stretching

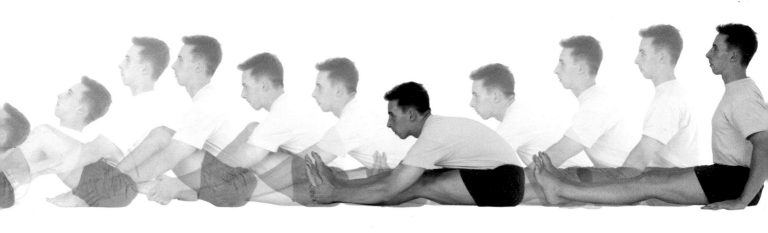

a *flow*motion™ title

stretching

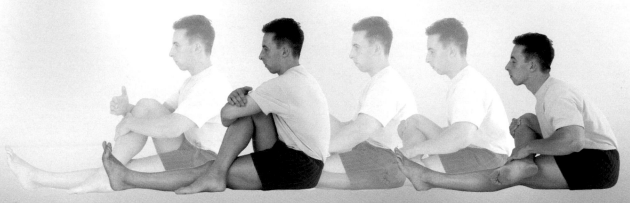

simon frost

Sterling Publishing Co., Inc.
New York

Created and conceived by
Axis Publishing Limited
8c Accommodation Road
London NW11 8ED
www.axispublishing.co.uk

Creative Director: Siân Keogh
Managing Editor: Matthew Harvey
Project Designer: Zöe Dissell
Project Editor: Michael Spilling
Production Manager: Sue Bayliss
Photographer: Mike Good

Library of Congress Cataloging-in-Publication
Data Available

10 9 8 7 6 5 4 3 2 1

Published in 2002 by Sterling Publishing Co., Inc.
387 Park Avenue South, New York, NY 10016
Text and images © Axis Publishing Limited 2002
Distributed in Canada by Sterling Publishing
c/o Canadian Manda Group,
One Atlantic Avenue, Suite 105
Toronto, Ontario, M6K 3E7, Canada

Separation by United Graphics Pte Limited
Printed and bound by Star Standard (Pte) Limited

Sterling ISBN 0–8069–8883–5

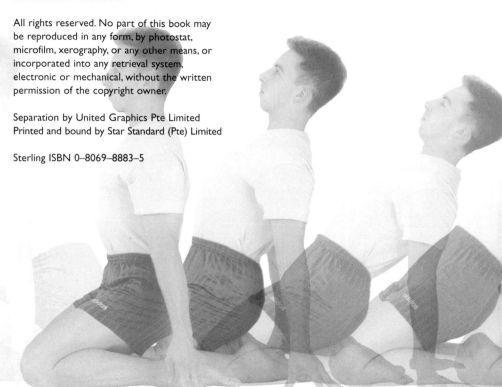

a *flow**motion*™ title
stretching

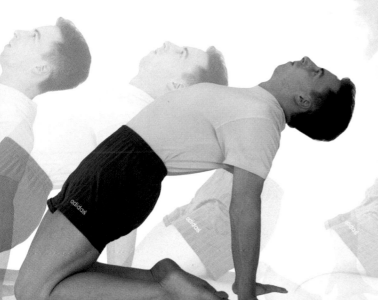

contents

introduction

This book is designed to provide a basic understanding of flexibility so that the reader can achieve a healthy flexibility that will improve their posture, fitness, and general well-being.

The aim of improved flexibility is to extend the range of movement (ROM) of our joints to the point where we are able to perform everyday activities with minimal effort and maximum effect. However, before we can reach this goal we should first understand what is meant by healthy flexibility. We will also look at the mechanics of flexibility, its limitations, and how it affects the functioning of our bodies.

healthy flexibility

Everyone should perform stretching exercises, whether or not they use it as a preparation for sports and other activities. Many people who do regular exercise tend to focus on their fitness, strength, and endurance and spend very little time improving their flexibility. Flexibility is one of the essential components of fitness because it improves performance and reduces muscular tension. An absence of stretching has been shown to increase the potential for injury through tight or stiff muscle fibers and create closed unhealthy postures.

Flexibility is specific to individual joints and the ability of those joints to move through their full ROM with little resistance from the surrounding muscle tissue. ROM varies from one joint to the next and according to the

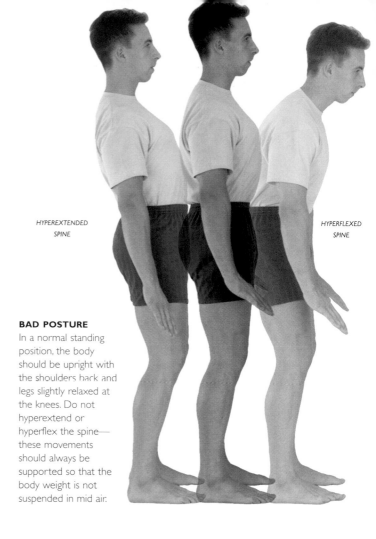

HYPEREXTENDED SPINE

HYPERFLEXED SPINE

BAD POSTURE
In a normal standing position, the body should be upright with the shoulders back and legs slightly relaxed at the knees. Do not hyperextend or hyperflex the spine—these movements should always be supported so that the body weight is not suspended in mid air.

kind of activity performed. Everyday living requires a certain ROM for healthy flexibility, while specific physical activities may need the ROM of particular joints to be much more flexible. The gains of flexibility are limited by a number of factors:

1. The elasticity of the connective tissue in and around the muscle fibers— that is, how elongated it can become and how it will progress over time.
2. The shape of the joint structure. For example, in hip abduction (raising the leg sideways), if the muscle tissue is highly elongated the ROM may be limited by the hip bones rather than the muscle resistance.
3. The ligaments that hold the bones together can also elongate to allow further movement in abduction, but may cause subluxion of the joint.
4. Genetics play a role in determining the bones' shape and the elasticity of the connective tissue.

static and dynamic training

There are two main types of flexibility training: static, which is when a muscle is held stretched for a length of time; and dynamic, which involves slow or fast movement into stretched positions, but which are not held. Static flexibility training concentrates on individual muscles and joints whereas dynamic training uses multiple muscles and joints combined with neuromuscular co-ordination and strength. Dynamic movements are important because they are specific to every day activity, but they risk a greater chance of injury due to the speed and force of the stretch.

THE BENEFITS OF FLEXIBILITY

IMPROVED MOVEMENT Flexibility can improve physical performance. As there is less tissue resistance, it requires less energy to achieve the ROM.
FEWER INJURIES With less tissue resistance there is a decreased chance of injury as you are less likely to exceed the tissue's extensibility during movements.
INCREASED BLOOD SUPPLY By moving joints through the full ROM, there is an increase in blood and nutrient supply to the joint structures, improving health and mobility.
IMPROVED JOINT STRENGTH Greater ROM exercise increases the quantity of synovial fluid (the protective lubricant that aids joint movement) and increases the viscosity of the fluid to allow greater and easier movement with more efficient nutrient transportation. An increase in synovial fluid may reduce the degeneration of joint structures, which can cause arthritic conditions.
BETTER MUSCLE COORDINATION Flexibility improves neuromuscular co-ordination. The time taken for messages to travel from the muscle to the brain is reduced due to the adaptation of the nervous tissue and its ability to isolate muscle response.
IMPROVED POSTURE AND BALANCE Flexibility training encourages better resting muscle tension to improve postural balance and awareness. It helps realign soft tissue structures that may have adapted to closed postural positions. Realignment reduces the effort needed to adopt good posture.
RELIEVES LOWER BACK PAIN Lower back pain can be reduced by an increase in lumbar and pelvic movement, which is improved by elongating the hamstrings, hip flexors, gluteals, and lumbar muscles.
RELIEVES MUSCLE STRESS Stretching is an excellent method of relieving muscular stress and mental tension. Tense muscles have reduced blood supply. They also have a greater toxicity that may cause lethargy. Better muscle equilibrium creates a sense of vitality and well-being.

too much of a good thing

While flexibility is a great asset to health and fitness, too much can be detrimental. Over flexibility within the joints is normally due to excessively elongated ligaments, which reduces joint stability and exposes the joint to injury. The amount of flexibility required depends on the activity. Excessive ROM without adequate muscle strength will increase the effect of degenerative disease and reduce the protective reflexes designed to avoid excessive movement. Some muscles may already be over flexible in relation to their opposing muscles. Many adults suffer from over flexibility due to excessive postures: for example, slouching over a desk may cause single joint structures to be placed in a prolonged stretch. With the effects of gravity and reduced muscle resistance, the body's posture may gradually adapt to that position. These muscles may develop a stretch weakness, which leave them vulnerable to injury even during mild movements.

A stretch weakness occurs when a muscle loses its elasticity through long-term postural deviation. For example, allowing the shoulders to slump forward can eventually feel comfortable. The weight of the limbs and reduced muscle resistance will have a greater downward force than the antagonistic muscles—the upper back muscles—that give resting recoil tension. Therefore, these muscles must be gently strengthened to slowly reduce flexibility and increase resting tension, while their antagonistic muscles—the chest and shoulders—must increase flexibility to reduce resting tension. This will result in the shoulders pulling upright to a correct posture, which will become the new comfort zone.

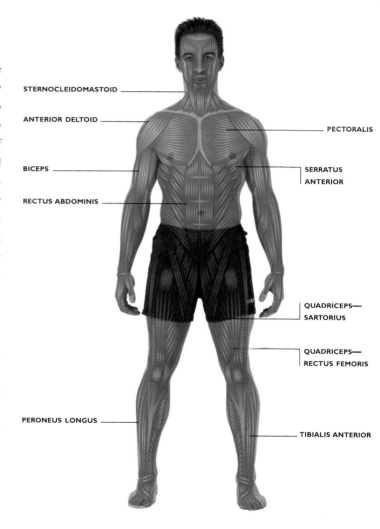

STERNOCLEIDOMASTOID

ANTERIOR DELTOID

PECTORALIS

BICEPS

SERRATUS ANTERIOR

RECTUS ABDOMINIS

QUADRICEPS— SARTORIUS

QUADRICEPS— RECTUS FEMORIS

PERONEUS LONGUS

TIBIALIS ANTERIOR

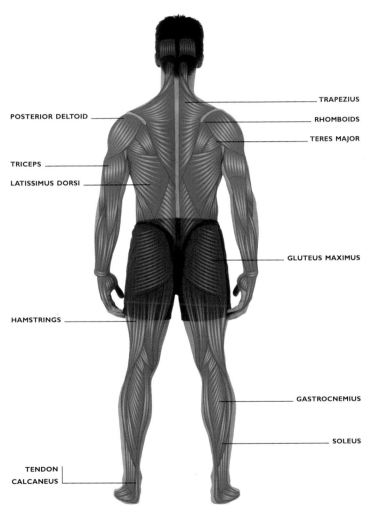

POSTERIOR DELTOID

TRICEPS

LATISSIMUS DORSI

HAMSTRINGS

TENDON
CALCANEUS

TRAPEZIUS

RHOMBOIDS

TERES MAJOR

GLUTEUS MAXIMUS

GASTROCNEMIUS

SOLEUS

muscle adaptation

We can improve flexibility through a wide variety of stretching methods. Generally, this is achieved by adding force to a muscle until it becomes stretched either passively or actively. The stretching sensation is caused in part by the connective tissue in and around the muscle involuntarily contracting against the applied force. The connective tissue is made of non-elastic collagen fibers and a small amount of elastic fibers that contain two mechanical properties.

ELASTIC ELONGATION occurs when muscle tissue is stretched and then released and then returned to its resting length once the force is removed. This application gives a temporary gain in flexibility in the same way that a spring will return to its original state once it is released from pressure. Stretching the elastic connective tissue is normally done with a high force, short duration technique called dynamic stretching.

PLASTIC ELONGATION is a more permanent change in length and tension. For example, if we take a piece of clay and pull it into a long string-like shape, it will not return to its original position unless physically manipulated. Plastic elongation occurs to non-elastic collagen fibers in the muscle and reforms them into a longer position. They will only shorten through muscular contractions without stretching—that is, any type of resistance training or cardiovascular exercise. A low force, long duration, static stretching technique is usually used to gain plastic deformation.

active and passive stretching

ACTIVE STRETCHING is the contraction of the antagonistic muscle to provide force against the stretched muscle. For example, when the leg is raised straight in front of the body, the quadriceps (at the front of the thigh) contract while the hamstrings (at the back of the thigh) become stretched. Active stretching strengthens the contracting muscles and reduces the stretch resistance of the elongated muscles. Active stretching is better with the dynamic technique (see page 9), although it does not lead to as much muscle development as the passive method. However, the combined use of strength with co-ordination is more common among sportspeople, who develop muscles for particular activities.

PASSIVE STRETCHING occurs when the muscle being stretched has an external force applied to it. For example, in an upright hamstring stretch, where the resting foot is place on an object of knee height or above, the

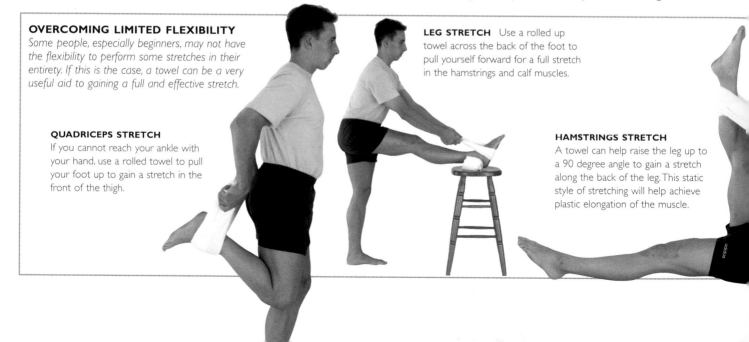

OVERCOMING LIMITED FLEXIBILITY
Some people, especially beginners, may not have the flexibility to perform some stretches in their entirety. If this is the case, a towel can be a very useful aid to gaining a full and effective stretch.

QUADRICEPS STRETCH
If you cannot reach your ankle with your hand, use a rolled towel to pull your foot up to gain a stretch in the front of the thigh.

LEG STRETCH Use a rolled up towel across the back of the foot to pull yourself forward for a full stretch in the hamstrings and calf muscles.

HAMSTRINGS STRETCH
A towel can help raise the leg up to a 90 degree angle to gain a stretch along the back of the leg. This static style of stretching will help achieve plastic elongation of the muscle.

force applied is the weight of the body leaning over the stretched leg. This does not require voluntary contractions in any of the muscles.

Sometimes it is better to stretch to gain both plastic (static/passive) and elastic (dynamic/active) elongation. For example, a martial arts expert is able to kick very high, the height of the kick being determined by the strength in the quadriceps and the stretch resistance in the hamstrings. If the expert were to use the static technique of stretching to achieve permanent elongation, the kick would become much higher with less risk of

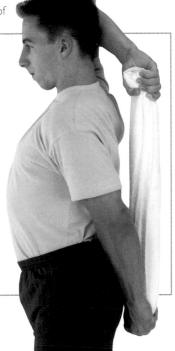

TRICEP STRETCH If you are unable to push your arm down between your shoulder blades, hold a towel in the raised hand, let it fall down the spine, then grasp the other end with the other hand. Now pull a stretch using the lower arm.

injury due to an increase in the tissue's extensibility. This would require less force from the working muscles. If the static technique were combined with the dynamic technique, a greater amount of strength and co-ordination would achieve a higher kick with less effort.

For good health we do not need this amount of ROM, but should have a good static flexibility. Beginners should aim for plastic elongation through static stretching until optimum movement is achieved. Only after having achieved the best you can from static movement is it advisable to improve dynamic flexibility (see Dynamic Stretches, pages 88–125).

tissue damage

When plastic elongation occurs there is some tissue damage, which can cause mild muscle soreness. The weakness is only short term while molecular reconstruction creates a new resting length for the muscle. For example, if we take a hot steel rod and pull both ends until it lengthens, the metal becomes weak at the point of elongation due to the molecular reconstruction. As the metal cools the strength is regained. Over-stretching can lead to serious tissue damage and reduce flexibility.

Another factor affecting elongation is temperature. When body temperature increases by just a few degrees, there is a reduced muscle resistance and greater muscle elasticity. A high force, short duration stretch at normal or above average temperatures will induce elastic elongation and a temporary gain in flexibility. Alternatively, a low force, long duration stretch at high temperatures will produce long-term plastic deformation.

the stretch reflex

The primary sensory organ in a muscle is called the muscle spindle. This allows muscles to sense and respond to a stretch. The muscle spindle sits parallel to the muscle fibers and measures the speed and force at which the stretch occurs. If the stretch is fast the spindle sends a signal to the spinal cord which returns with a message causing the stretched muscle to contract and resist the direction of movement. This is a protective response to inhibit extreme movement at high velocity. The spindle halts activation when the force is revoked by sending a message to the spinal cord to relax the contracted muscle. An example of this is the snapping back of the head when falling asleep sitting upright. The sudden relaxation of the neck muscles and the combined effects of gravity allow the head to drop quickly into a stretch, firing the muscle spindle mechanism and lifting the head. By regularly exercising the muscle spindle, it will become less sensitive to force and allow greater movement at higher velocities.

The secondary sensory organ is called the gorgi tendon organ (GTO). This is much less sensitive than the spindle reflex and is fired when the spindle and muscles are overloaded to

FLEXION AND EXTENSION Flexion describes bending or decreasing the angle at a joint, while extension describes straightening or increasing the angle. All the major joints—the hips, knees, shoulders, wrists, and elbows—can be flexed and extended.

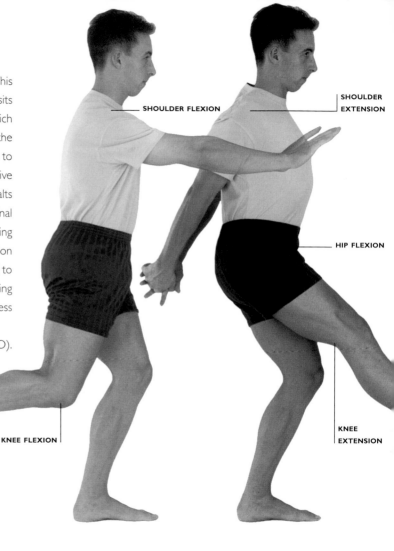

SHOULDER FLEXION

SHOULDER EXTENSION

HIP FLEXION

KNEE FLEXION

KNEE EXTENSION

the point where there is a risk of muscle rupture. When this occurs the GTO overrides the impulses of the spindle, causing the muscle to relax, but opens the joint structure to potential damage. For this reason, avoid applying too much force to the muscle, as each time the GTO is used it becomes less sensitive and risks possible muscle rupture.

pulsing

To manipulate the muscle spindle, use small, slow, controlled pulses to gain further elongation. At the point of mild stretch, a releasing sensation can be felt if the position is held for a long enough period of time. At this point, slightly release the tension and cease the spindle reflex. The muscle fibers relax, making it possible to pulse and hold a slightly more elongated state before the spindle is re-fired. This process is called pulsing, and will allow you to hold and extend a stretch.

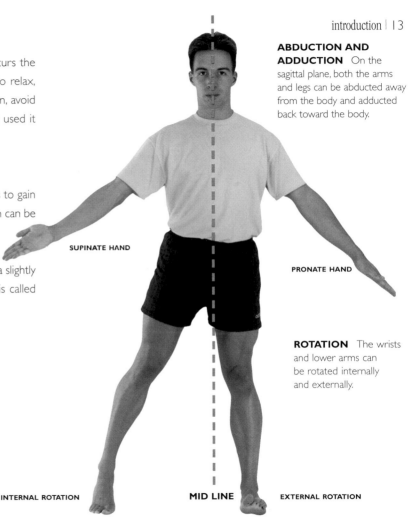

ABDUCTION AND ADDUCTION On the sagittal plane, both the arms and legs can be abducted away from the body and adducted back toward the body.

SUPINATE HAND

PRONATE HAND

ROTATION The wrists and lower arms can be rotated internally and externally.

PLANTARFLEXION

FLEXING THE FEET Unlike the knee and elbow joints, the feet can be flexed in two directions—dorsiflexion, to bring the foot up, and plantarflexion, to bring the toes down.

INTERNAL ROTATION

MID LINE

EXTERNAL ROTATION

factors affecting flexibility workouts

HEAT This is an important factor for muscle elongation. A good way to gain maximum potential for development is to take a warm bath and then stretch in a warm room. Another effective method is to stretch after aerobic exercise, increasing the core temperature of the muscle.

COMFORT To relax effectively you need to feel at ease

ANXIETY Worry and anxiety may be detrimental to the stretch reflex.

The chart below outlines how each section of the book may be used to gain the most out of flexibility training. The *Flowmotion* illustrations demonstrate a full health-related ROM and it is not advisable to push flexibility further unless for sports specific purposes. Once you have achieved full health-related postures, you can progress to the final section, Dynamic Stretches (see pages 88–125), to improve strength and endurance, co-ordination, relaxation, and general well-being.

AIM	HEALTH, FITNESS AND FLEXIBILITY; POST-EXERCISE FLEXIBILITY	DYNAMIC STRETCHES— MAINTENANCE AND DEVELOPMENT	PRE-EXERCISE STRETCHING	BACK STRETCHES— DEVELOPMENTAL STRETCHING
FREQUENCY	3–6 times per week	3–5 times per week	done before any sport or exercise activity	daily; in severe cases to be done 2–3 times a day
INTENSITY	low force, long duration stretching	high force, short duration stretching	medium force, short duration stretching	low force medium duration stretching
TIME	General workout will vary from 10–40 minutes; stretch positions should be held for 15–30 seconds between pulses.	General workout time will be anywhere from 15–20 minutes; stretch positions will not be held for any length of time.	Hold stretches for 15–30 seconds; general workout should take no longer than 3 minutes.	Hold for 15–30 seconds; general workout should take anywhere from 10 minutes upwards.
TYPE	static stretching, passively applied force for plastic elongation	dynamic stretching, actively applied force using muscle strength	static, elastic elongation, passively applied force	static, plastic elongation with passively applied force
NOTES	Allow adequate recovery between sessions. Hold the stretch until a release in tension occurs. Small, slow and controlled pulses are best. In post exercise this should be done to reduce stiffness.	Movements should be slow and controlled, taken to full ROM and repeated between 6–10 times each session.	Stretches can combine muscles to save time. They should only be repeated once, in order to gain elastic elongation to minimize injury prior to exercise.	Movements should be slow and controlled and taken to the point of mild tension. No pulsing— repeat for development.

go with the flow

The special *Flowmotion* images used in this book have been created to ensure that you see the whole stretch—not just selected highlights. Each of the image sequences flow across the page from left to right, demonstrating how the stretch progresses and how to get into each position safely and effectively. Each stretch is labelled as being suitable for beginners,

intermediate, or advanced students by a colored tab above the title. The captions along the bottom of the images provide additional information to help you perform the stretches confidently. Below this, another layer of information is contained in the timeline, including instructions for breathing and symbols indicating when to hold a position.

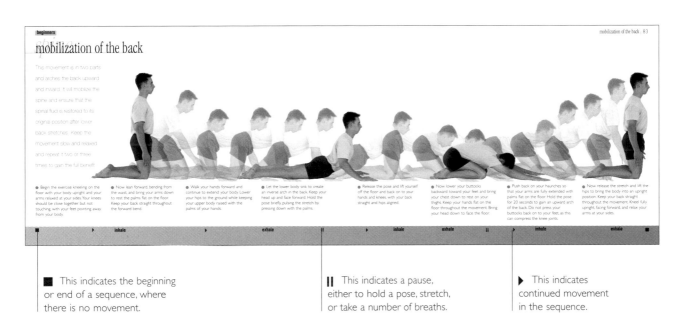

■ This indicates the beginning or end of a sequence, where there is no movement.

‖ This indicates a pause, either to hold a pose, stretch, or take a number of breaths.

▶ This indicates continued movement in the sequence.

health, fitness, and flexibility

lying hamstring stretch

hamstrings and hips

This is a progressive exercise that stretches the hamstrings (the biceps femoris, semitendinosus, and semimembranosus) by extending the legs to an upright position. The hamstrings are one of the main muscles that extend the thigh and leg.

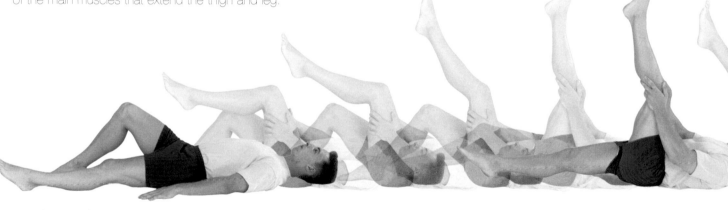

● Lie flat on the floor with your feet extended and relaxed. Raise your right leg so that the sole of the foot is resting on the floor and the knee is bent at a 90 degree angle. This will be your supporting leg.

● Now slowly raise your left leg, using your hands to help move your thigh back toward your chest and into an upright position. Keep your head relaxed and on the floor throughout the movement.

● Slowly straighten your left leg in a gentle movement, sliding your hands up toward your calf as the leg extends. Keep your right leg bent to avoid straining your hamstring or lower back.

● Gently extend your left leg until it is pointing upright. The raise will also put pressure on your lower back—to avoid the vertebrae becoming compressed, do not allow your bottom to lift from the floor.

■   inhale   ▶   exhale   ▌▌

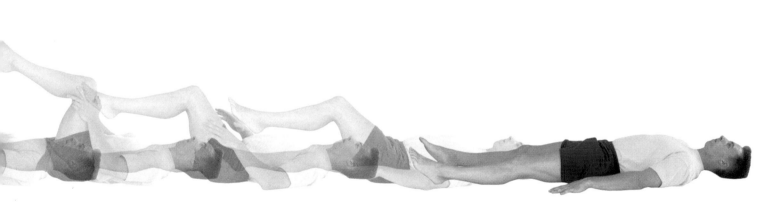

● Lower and fully extend your right leg to rest gently on the floor. You will feel a stretch along the back of your left thigh, and around your right hip. Beginners often over-extend—if you feel pain in your extended leg, bend at the knee to relieve the pressure.

● To come out of the stretch, reverse the process by gently lowering the leg and allowing the hands to slide down from the calf to the thigh. Remember not to raise your back from the floor.

● Continue to lower your left leg until it is resting flat on the floor. Relax and breathe deeply. Now repeat the stretch with the other leg.

● If you wish to achieve a greater stretch, use a rolled towel around the ankle of the raised leg and pull when the leg is fully extended. Beginners can also use the rolled towel to achieve a stretch without compromising the correct posture.

▶ inhale　　　▶ exhale　　　■

standing hamstring stretch *hips*

This is a progressive movement that targets the hamstrings and hips. It is more advanced than the Lying Hamstring Stretch (see pages 18–19) and should only be attempted by those who have been practicing stretching for some time.

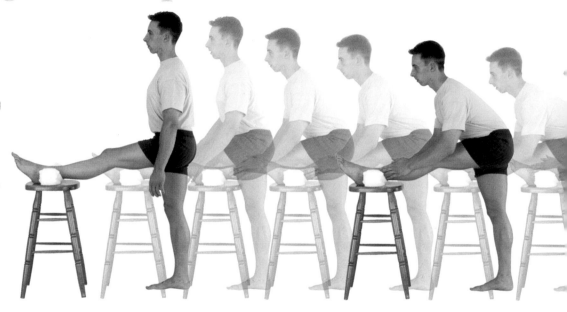

● To perform this exercise, you will need a stool (or similar item) on which to rest your foot and a rolled-up towel to provide support for your ankle. The stool should be roughly waist height. You may also want to stand near a wall for support.

● Place your weaker leg on the stool with the towel supporting your ankle. Your heel should be resting on the surface of the stool. Your leg can be slightly bent or straight, depending on your flexibility.

● Keep your standing leg "soft" and do not lock at the knee. Keep your hips square throughout the exercise to avoid putting pressure on the lower back. Place your hands on either side of your extended knee.

● Flexing from the waist, slowly bend your body forward, sliding your hands along the leg. Your back should be straight throughout the movement.

inhale ▶ ▶ **exhale** ▶

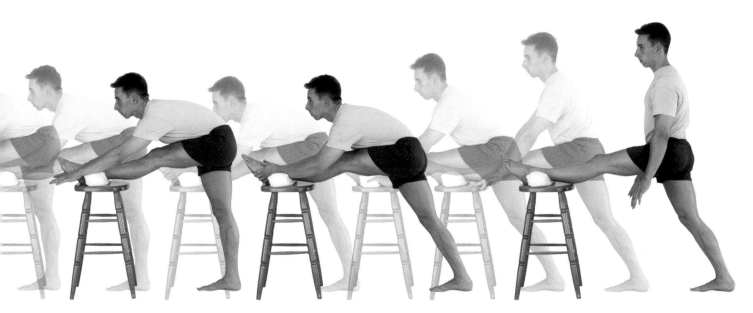

● Keeping your hips square, continue to bend forward until your hands reach your ankle. If you are flexible enough, extend your arms beyond the ankle to rest your forearms on the towel. Hold the pose.

● You will feel a stretch along your hamstring and in your arms as you fully extend. You will also feel a slight stretch in your lower back, which is allowed to arch slightly at the furthest point of the extension.

● Now slowly reverse the movement, raising up from the waist and sliding your hands back along the leg to return to the start position. Repeat the stretch on the other leg.

● For a more extreme stretch, when your are fully extended, shuffle your standing leg away from the stool. To dismount from the stool, shuffle your standing leg forward and bend your outstretched leg until you can easily reach the stool with your hands.

ll   **inhale and exhale**   ▶   **inhale**   ▶   **exhale**   **ll**

kneeling hip flexor and quadriceps

This exercise is a progressive movement that offers beginners positions and advanced variations to increase the stretch in the quadriceps (anterior thigh) and hip flexors. Perform this exercise on a soft surface to avoid damaging the knee joints.

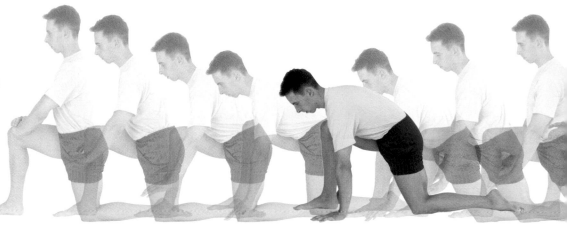

● Begin the exercise with your left leg kneeling on the floor, and your right leg bent at the knee forming a 90 degree angle to the body. Use your hands to push on the right leg to ensure that the head and body are held upright.

● Keeping your hips facing forward and stomach tucked in, slowly extend your arms forward and allow the fingers to slide along the floor until the palms are pronate. At the same time, extend your left leg away from the body, sliding the toes along the floor.

● With palms pressed firmly against the floor, gently pulse the left leg to feel a stretch in the upper thigh. Make sure that the hips remain square and facing forward during the stretch, otherwise, the back will arch.

● Release the stretch and bring your extended arms back into the body. Place your hands back on the right leg. Keep the left leg extended, with the knee resting on the floor. Check that your head and body are upright and the chest is pushed out.

■   inhale ▶   exhale   ‖   inhale ▶

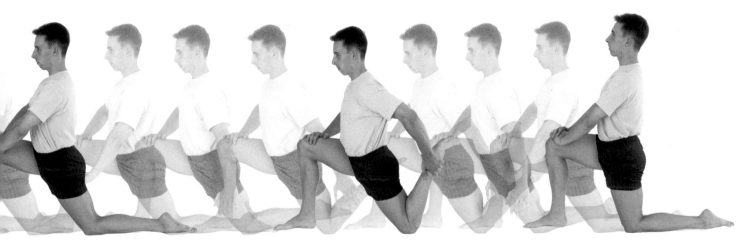

● To move into the advanced position, slowly raise the left foot to within three inches (eight centimeters) of the body; any closer will compress the knee joint. Using the right leg and arm to support the body, grasp the left ankle with the left hand.

● Pull gently on the foot to extend the stretch and then release. This advanced stretch works the quad muscles when the leg is drawn toward the body. Check that your hips are held square with the body to prevent the back from slouching.

● Release your grip on the left ankle and allow the foot to return to the floor. Slowly bring the extended leg into the body, sliding the foot along the floor. Bring the left arm to the front of the body and rest the hand behind the knee of the right leg.

● Use the arms to push against the right leg and restore the upright head and body pose. This exercise can be repeated on alternate legs until you find it difficult to push yourself away from the floor and back into the original kneeling position.

▶ **exhale**   ‖   ▶   ■

standing quadriceps stretch

This exercise stretches the quadriceps (the anterior thigh muscles). The quadriceps rectus femoris extends the leg and is the largest muscle in the body. Beginners might find it helpful to use a rolled-up towel to help raise the foot.

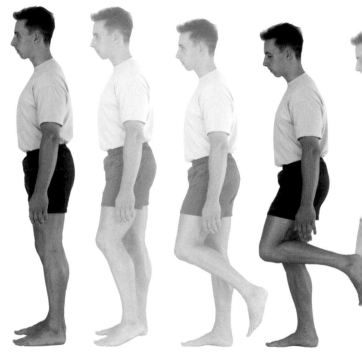

● Stand upright with arms and legs relaxed. Your knees should be quite close together—approximately a hand's width apart.

● Now slowly flex your left knee and raise your left ankle toward your buttocks while maintaining balance on your standing leg. If you find balancing on one leg difficult, stand near a wall and use your right arm for support.

● Continue to raise your foot while slowly bringing your left hand back to meet the foot. Hold the foot just below the ankle.

● Pull the ankle back slightly, but do not bring it back to touch the buttocks, as this can compress the knee joint. Keep your balancing leg slightly bent and soft at the knee—do not lock the knee joint.

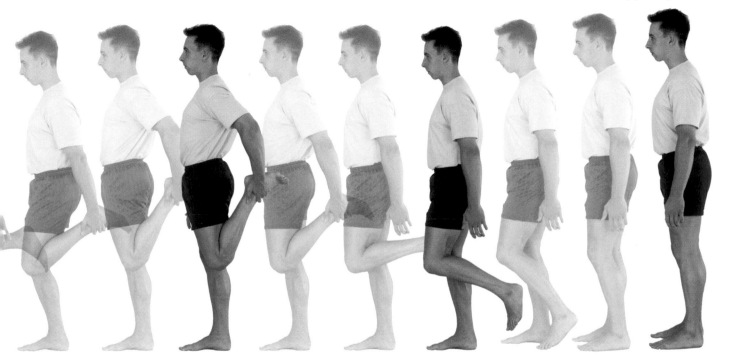

● To complete the stretch, cup the ankle with your left hand and push your hips slightly forward. Adjust your body weight on to your right leg, push your chest forward, and pull gently on the leg with your left hand.

● Breathe deeply and hold this position, but do not pull the heel into the buttocks, as this can compress the knee joint. You will feel a stretch down the front of your upper thigh and hip.

● Now gently release your ankle and lower the leg to floor. Return your hands to your sides, put your left foot flat on the floor, and redistribute your body weight evenly.

● Now perform the movement on the other leg. Remember that if you cannot easily reach your ankle, you can use a towel wrapped around the ankle to help raise the foot.

exhale   ❙❙   ▶   breathe normally   ▶   ■

standing calf stretch
gastrocnemius and soleus

This is a progressive exercise that stretches the gastrocnemius and soleus muscles in the calves. Both muscles are used in plantarflexing the ankle joint. The sequence stretches the calves on the left leg then those on the right in turn.

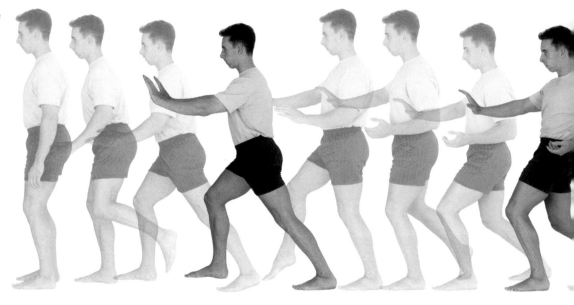

● Stand facing a wall with your knees relaxed. Now slowly raise your left leg and step it backward, making sure that the standing leg bears the main part of your body weight.

● Press the heel of your left leg down toward the floor to gain a full extension. Simultaneously, raise your hands toward the wall.

● Keep your resting leg bent at the knee, but do not allow the knee joint to extend beyond the end of your right toes. For correct posture, keep your hips square, chest forward, and head up throughout the movement.

● Progress the stretch by pressing your palms against the wall and pushing. Hold the pose and feel a stretch along the upper part of the calf muscles (the gastrocnemius muscle) in the back of your left leg.

■　　　▶ **inhale**　　　**exhale**　Ⅱ　**inhale**　　　▶ **exhale**

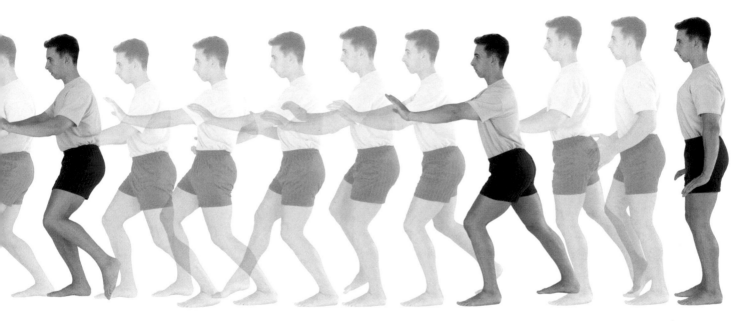

● To attain a full stretch, you will need to remove your hands from the wall and ease your body weight back onto your left leg. You will feel an additional stretch at the lower end of the calf, in the soleus muscle.

● Now step your body back to the starting position so that you can perform the stretch on the opposite leg. Shift your weight to your left leg and step your right leg backward.

● Remember not to allow your resting knee joint to extend beyond your toes. Keep your hips square and chest forward throughout the movement. Fully extend the right leg and complete the stretch.

● Return to the standing upright position. Finish the exercise with your knees relaxed and your hands resting at your sides.

ll	**inhale**	▶	**exhale**	▶ ■

seated adductor stretch

This is a flowing movement that stretches the adductor muscles (the longus, brevis, and magnus) along the insides of the thighs. The adductors are the muscles that we use to bring the legs together. They work with the abductors—the muscles on the outside that open the legs.

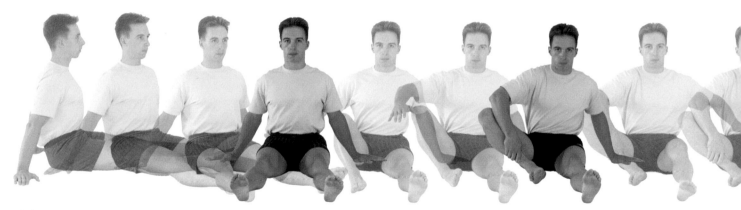

● Sit with your legs extended in front and your hands behind you with your palms resting flat on the floor. Press your hands flat against the floor to support the body.

● Push your chest out, keep your back straight, and keep your elbows soft and do not allow them to lock.

● Now slowly bend your right leg and bring it in toward the center line of the body. Grip your shin with your right hand to guide the leg inward while maintaining stability using your resting hand.

● Once the right leg is tucked in, use your left hand to help guide your left leg in toward the center line. Place the soles of your feet together.

inhale ▶ **exhale** ▶ **inhale** ▶

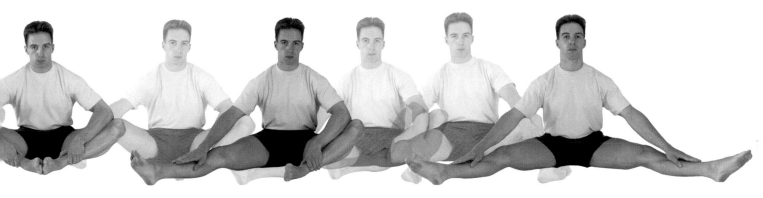

● Now press down with your arms to move your knees apart. Keep your back straight and do not lean forward, as this can strain your lower back. You will feel a stretch along the insides of your thighs. Hold the pose.

● Keeping your back upright and straight, slowly guide your right leg with your hand facing outward and fully extend at a 45 degree angle. Rest your right hand on your shin.

● Do the same with your left leg and rest your left hand on your shin. Point your toes outward and stretch your legs as far they will go. If your lower back lacks flexibility, use your arms to press your legs wider apart to achieve a full stretch.

● Keeping your back upright and shoulders back, breathe deeply and hold the stretch. Release the stretch and bring the legs together again.

‖ inhale   ▶ exhale   ▶ ‖

seated hip rotators *lower back and hamstrings*

This is a more difficult exercise that will test the adductor muscles on the insides of the thighs as well as stretch the lower back and hamstrings. You will need good spinal flexibility to perform this sequence.

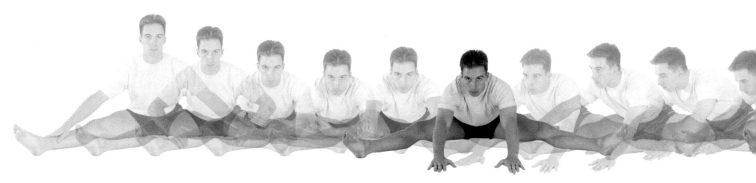

● Begin the exercise sitting on the floor with your feet extended in front of you (in the finishing posture of the Adductor Stretch on pages 28–29). Throughout this exercise your lower spine should be upright to avoid slumping and straining the muscles.

● To perform the first stage, slowly lean forward and push your arms out in front of you, flexing from the lower waist. Push your hands forward and not downward toward the floor.

● Push out a far as you can to achieve a good stretch on the inner thighs. Do not let your feet rotate inward when stretching. Now use your left hand to lead the body into a sideways rotation.

● Bring your right arm to the outside of your right leg and reach forward to grasp the sole of the foot. Stretch the body sideways so that your fingers are about two inches (six centimeters) from the foot, but not touching.

| ■ | **inhale** | ▶ | **‖ exhale and inhale** | ▶ | **exhale** | ▶ |

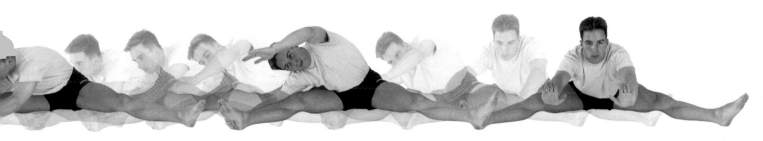

● At full stretch, your body should be virtually square with the floor. Hold the position and feel a stretch in the hamstrings of your right leg and your lower back.

● Now pull your body away from your extended leg and rotate to the left from the waist. Using the same technique, stretch your arms to the left. You will feel a stretch in your hamstrings and lower back.

● Raise your body from the sideways rotation and lean forward, reaching with both arms to stretch your lower back and adductors. Again, push outward as far as you can without letting your feet turn inward.

● Finish the exercise by raising your body back to the start position, keeping your back straight throughout. Relax and rest your hands.

‖   inhale   ▶   ‖   exhale   inhale   ▶   exhale   ‖

lower back progressed *and lumbar vertebrae*

This is a good introductory exercise that will stretch the lower back, lumbar spine, and hamstring muscles. Do not attempt the second part of this exercise if you suffer from muscular back pain. For the hamstring stretch, you can use a rolled up towel to support the underside of the knee. This will ensure that the center of the muscle is stretched, and not the ligaments.

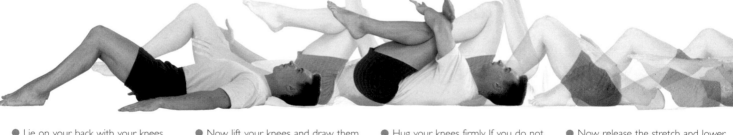

● Lie on your back with your knees raised and the soles of your feet pressed flat on the floor. Your knees should be bent to roughly 90 degrees. Your hands should be flat at your sides with the palms facing downward.

● Now lift your knees and draw them in toward your chest. Bring your arms up and wrap them around your knees, hugging your knees into your chest.

● Hug your knees firmly. If you do not feel any tension in the back, progress the exercise by hugging more tightly to gain a full squeeze that will eject any excess air. This should be a quick effortless movement to avoid putting pressure on the lower back.

● Now release the stretch and lower your knees down to the start position to bring the soles of your feet to rest flat on the ground.

| ■ inhale ▶ | exhale ❚❚ ▶ inhale ▶ |

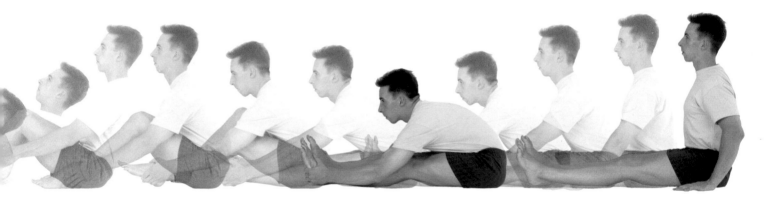

● Now raise your upper body from the waist. Stretch your arms forward as you perform this movement to provide balance. Reach forward with your hands toward your feet.

● With your body fully upright, grasp the soles of your feet and walk them forward until your legs are fully extended and flat on the floor. Keep your head facing forward throughout the forward bend.

● Keep your toes pointed toward the sky. Pulse the stretch as far as you can without causing discomfort. You will feel a stretch in your lower back and in the hamstring muscles. To avoid discomfort, you can rest the hollow of the knee on a rolled up towel.

● Release the stretch and lean back to sit upright with your head facing forward. Place your hands at your sides and rest your palms flat on the floor. Relax and breathe deeply.

begin to exhale ▶ ‖ exhale ▶ ■

disc energizer *spinal flexibility*

This exercise helps to move fluid around the spine, promoting good alignment, balance, and increased mobilization. Remember to perform the stretch on both sides to balance the spinal fluid.

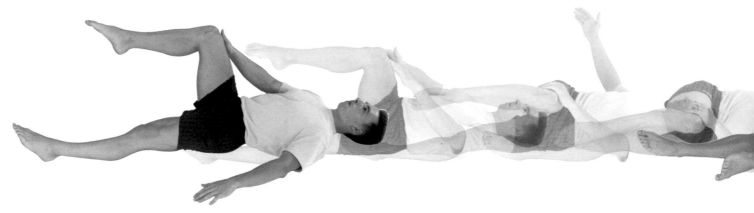

● Begin this exercise lying flat on your back with your feet spread roughly shoulder width apart. Place your arms flat on the floor, away from your sides with your palms facing downward.

● Slowly lift your right knee up to 90 degrees while raising your right hand to rest on the knee. Keep your body straight and back flat against the floor throughout this movement.

● Now turn your right knee to the left, using your right hand to guide it over your left leg. Turn from the hips, not the lower spine. Keep your left leg extended throughout the movement.

● Continue to bring the knee down toward the floor, rolling your hips to the left as you do so. It is safe to roll the hips in this exercise because both feet are off the floor, avoiding any unnecessary compression on the back.

■ ▶ **inhale** ▶ **exhale** ▶

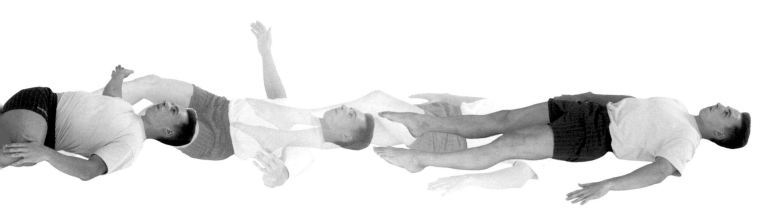

● Once your right leg is across the left leg, use the left hand to pull the knee down to rest on the floor. Stretch your right arm in the opposite direction to ensure that your shoulders maintain contact with the floor throughout the stretch.

● Hold the stretch, keeping your knee bent at 90 degrees and your head and chest facing upward.

● Now release the stretch and bring the leg away from the floor, using your left hand to guide it over your body. Extend your right leg to lie flat and bring your arms down to your sides to return to the starting position.

● Now perform the stretch on the other side. If you experience any difference in mobility this may be due to the spinal fluid having moved to the opposite side. Perform the stretch slowly to allow time for the spinal fluid to rebalance itself.

‖　　　▶　　　**inhale**　　　▶　　　**exhale**　■

lying gluteal twist

glutals and lower back

This two-part exercise will stretch the gluteal muscles (the maximus, medius, and minimus) in the buttocks. The gluteal muscles are used to extend and abduct the thighs and stabilize the hip joints.

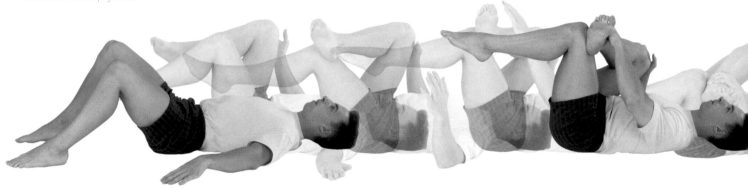

● Lie on your back with your knees raised and your feet flat on the floor and your arms rested at your sides.

● Now slowly raise your left leg to 90 degrees. Bring your right leg over your left knee, and as you do so, rotate your hips to the right. Rotate your right foot and guide the leg across with the right hand.

● Now grasp your right foot with your left hand and gently pull the body into a roll to the opposite side. The sole of your right foot should now rest flat on the floor. Hold your foot in position.

● Use your right knee to pull your foot back toward your face. Only pull the leg as far as it feels comfortable to do so. Do not lift your head or neck toward your knee as this could strain your neck and will undermine the effectiveness of the stretch.

begin to inhale ▶ **inhale** ▶ **begin to exhale** ▶

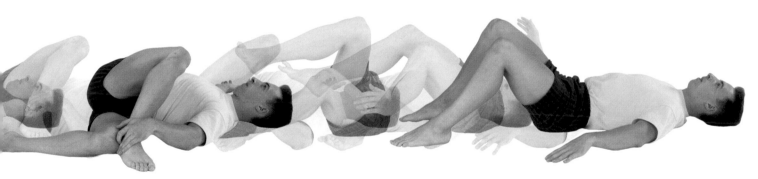

● Bring your right arm back to keep your shoulders flat against the floor. You will feel a stretch down the outside of your right buttock.

● Now roll your body back to the center, using your right arm to maintain balance. Roll your body quite quickly, and keep your right heel resting in the groove between the kneebone and the top of the thigh—a lower position will compress the knee.

● Hold the pose and feel a stretch along your right buttock. To increase the stretch, pulse the knee further.

● Now slowly lower your legs toward the floor, releasing your heel as soon as the pressure from the knee is removed. Place both feet on the floor and relax your arms at your sides. Now repeat the exercise with the other leg.

exhale   inhale   ▶   ‖   exhale   ◼

seated gluteal stretch

gluteus maximus

This is a progressive exercise that stretches the gluteal muscles in the buttocks. This stretch can help ease lower back tension, as the gluteals can compress the spine when they grow stiff.

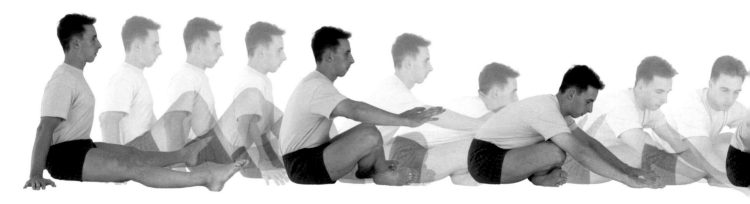

● Begin this exercise sitting upright with your legs extended, your spine straight and the palms of your hands resting flat on the floor at your sides.

● Using your hands to brace your body, lift your buttocks slightly off the floor and bring both legs toward your body to cross. You legs do not need to be in tight to the body. Keep your body upright and straight.

● Now push your hands forward, bending your back from the waist. Keep your arms roughly in line with your knees as you reach forward. Exhale deeply to help push the body down and reach your hands toward the floor, placing them palms down.

● Now turn your body to the right, rotating from the waist. Remember not to let your buttocks lift from the floor. Bend so that your head is in line with your knee. Place your right hand flat on the floor to support the body and stretch downward.

■   inhale   ▶   exhale   ‖   inhale   ▶

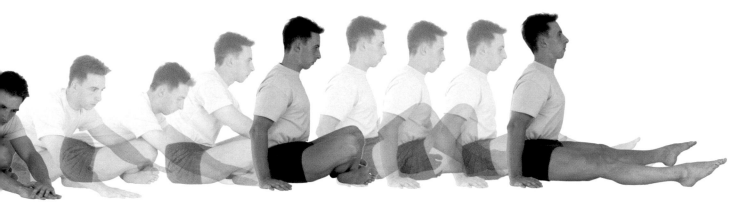

● Hold the stretch and pulse the movement. You will feel a stretch in your left gluteal muscle and a gentler stretch in your lower back.

● Now rotate your body back to face forward, keeping your arms stretched and your hands pressed on the ground throughout. Once you are facing forward again, lift your body up from the forward bend.

● Bring your head and back upright and place the palms of your hands flat on the floor at your sides. Using your hands to brace your body, lift your buttocks slightly off the floor and uncross your legs.

● Now extend your legs in front of you and point your toes forward, keeping your back upright. Now perform the stretch on the other side. If you feel the stretch is greater in one gluteal muscle than in the other, you may need to recross your legs.

‖　　　　　exhale　　　　▶　　　inhale　　　　　▶

standing lateral stretch

latissimus dorsi

This exercise involves a progressive, flowing movement that mobilizes the spine and stretches the latissimus dorsi. It is a good preparatory stretch for the Standing Rotation routine on pages 88–89.

● Stand with your feet roughly shoulder width apart and your arms hanging loosely at your sides. Keep your legs soft at the knees.

● Inhale and slowly raise your arms, crossing them as they pass in front of your chest. Move the arms in an upward movement that expands outward from the center.

● You should be fully inhaled as your hands reach head height. With your palms facing outward, extend your hands toward the sky, facing your head forward as you do. Exhale as your hands reach skyward.

● Lean to your left, flexing from the waist. Grasp your right wrist with your left hand to help pull your body downward. You should pull slightly to the front of your head, so that you can see the clasped hands above you.

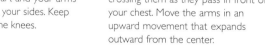

inhale ▶ exhale ‖ inhale ▶

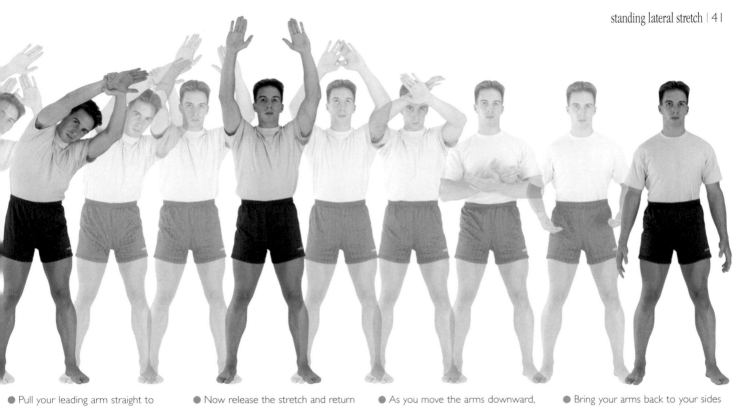

● Pull your leading arm straight to gain an elbow extension. You will feel a stretch in your latissimus dorsi muscles. If you find your hips are starting to move, you are leaning too far and should adjust your position.

● Now release the stretch and return the body to the center in an upright position with hands parted and stretching skyward. Now reverse the downward movement, exhale, and slowly lower your arms, again crossing them as they pass your chest.

● As you move the arms downward, keep them close to the body. Focus on pulling the hands downward and crossing them in front of your chest in a single flowing movement.

● Bring your arms back to your sides and relax your body. Now perform the stretch with the other arm.

❚❚   exhale   ▶   inhale   ▶   exhale   ■

back and chest stretch

rhomboids, pectoralis, anterior deltoids

This warm-up routine consists of two movements and will mobilize the rhomboid muscle (upper back), the pectoralis muscles (chest), and anterior deltoids (shoulders). To gain a good stretch, hold each position for between 15 and 20 seconds.

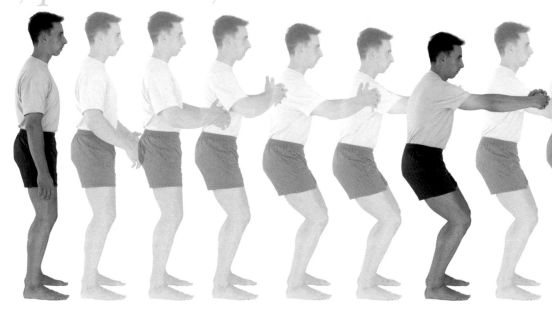

● Begin the exercise in the standing position, with your feet spaced no more than shoulder width apart. Keep the knees soft and make sure that they do not lock during the stretch. Your arms should be at your sides and the body held upright.

● Slowly bend both arms at the elbows and raise them until they are level with your waist. Bring the hands together in front of the body and interlock your fingers so that the hands are firmly clasped together with thumbs pointing upward.

● Raise your arms to chest height and extend them away from the body, letting the upper body lean forward slightly to create a stretch in the back. Bend the knees and push your bottom out from the midline as if you were about to sit.

● With your hips square, keep the body and arms forward and push the bottom out further to arch the back outward. To increase the stretch, lean lower and raise the arms higher. Now exhale and dip the body lower to pulse the movement.

■   **begin to inhale**   ▶   **inhale**   ▶   **II**

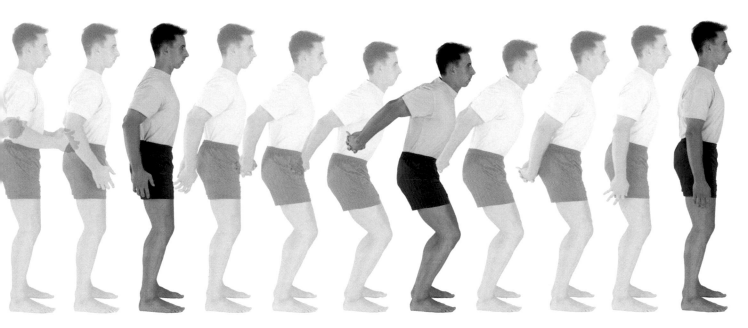

● Release the stretch and bring your clasped hands into the chest, then lower them to waist height. Unlock your fingers and let the arms slowly return to your sides. Check that both feet are facing forward.

● Now take your arms behind the body and clasp the hands together by interlocking your fingers. Bend the knees gently, and lean the upper body forward. Remember to keep the back straight as the body lowers; otherwise, the stretch in the chest will be lost.

● Push your buttocks away from the midline. Raise the arms to feel a stretch across the chest; you will feel a stretch in the front of the shoulders too as the arms get higher. At full stretch, exhale then bend forward to pulse the movement.

● Release the stretch and bring the arms back toward the body. Unclasp the hands and let them fall to the sides. Gently straighten the body into the upright position, making sure that the hips are square, the chest is pushed out, and the head is held up.

exhale ▶ inhale ▶ exhale ❚❚ ■

chest and triceps stretch *pectoralis*

triceps and pectoralis

This simple warm-up routine will stretch the pectoralis (chest) muscles and triceps along the back of the upper arm. For the triceps stretch, if you find it difficult to bend your arm behind your head, hold a rolled towel with the raised arm and pull on the other end with your resting arm.

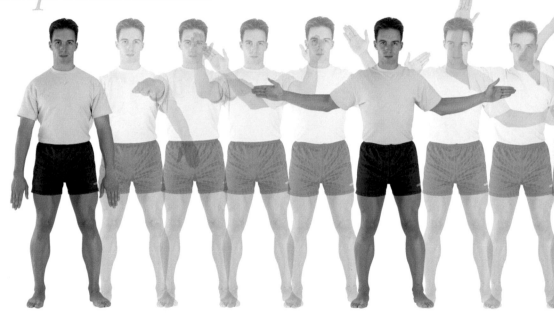

● Stand upright with your feet positioned shoulder width apart and your arms relaxed at your sides with your palms facing backward.

● Slowly raise your arms out in front, keeping your arms straight but not locked at the elbows. Bring the arms up to shoulder height so that they are parallel with the floor. Keep your knees relaxed throughout the exercise.

● Now push your arms out to the sides of the body so that the palms are facing forward and the elbows are slightly behind the body. Keep the elbows down when doing the stretch, otherwise the muscles in the shoulder joints could become trapped.

● Push the elbows and hands back to gain a stretch across the chest. Pulse the stretch for 10–20 seconds. You will feel a stretch across the chest.

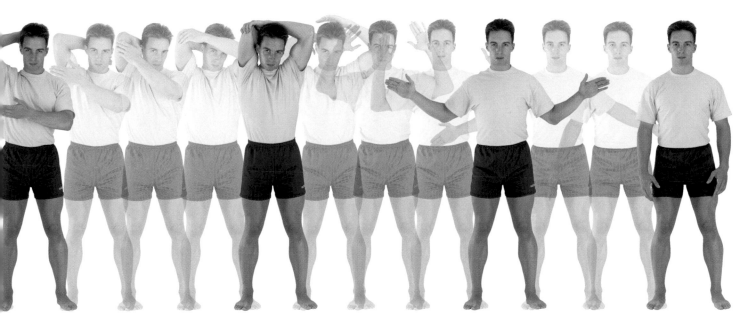

● Now raise your right arm and bring the hand and forearm behind your head so that the elbow is at 90 degrees. Bring your left hand up and over the top of your head to pull the right elbow to point vertically.

● Hold your elbow against your head with your hand resting downward between your shoulder blades. You will feel a stretch along your right triceps. Pulse the stretch for 20 seconds, pressing with the left arm to maintain the pressure.

● Release the stretch and bring both arms down and in front of your chest. Now bring your elbows out to your sides, keeping them below shoulder height with the palms facing outward. Repeat the chest stretch for 20 seconds, pulsing the movement.

● Now release the stretch and bring your arms back to your sides. For a more intense single arm chest stretch, you can place your hand against a wall with the arm bent at 90 degrees, then slowly turn the body away from the wall to extend the stretch.

inhale   ▶   exhale   ❚❚   inhale   ▶   ■

standing neck stretch

This is a good pre-exercise warm-up that can be performed in just a few minutes. The movement will stretch your neck muscles (the sternocleidomastoid and trapezius) and relieve tension in the shoulders and neck.

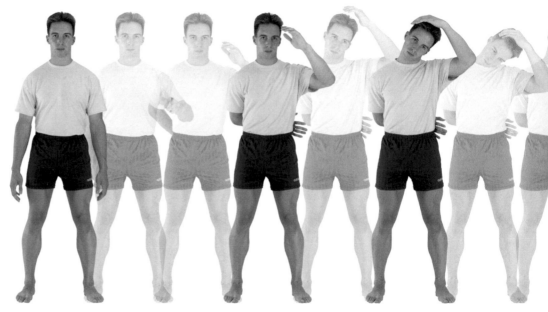

● This is a tension-relieving movement that rounds off the opening routine to remove any stress that has built up. For this reason, the routine does not need to be progressed for a more intense stretch.

● Stand upright with your feet positioned shoulder width apart and your arms relaxed at your sides with your palms facing behind you.

● Raise your left hand up toward your head and move your right arm behind your back so that the elbow is at 90 degrees and the forearm is resting in the small of your back. Bring your raised hand over your head to grasp the right side of your crown.

● Relax your neck muscles and gently pull down with the hand, keeping your body upright. Do not pull your whole upper body, but keep the movement isolated to the neck.

■   ❙❙   **begin to inhale**   ▶   **inhale**   ❙❙

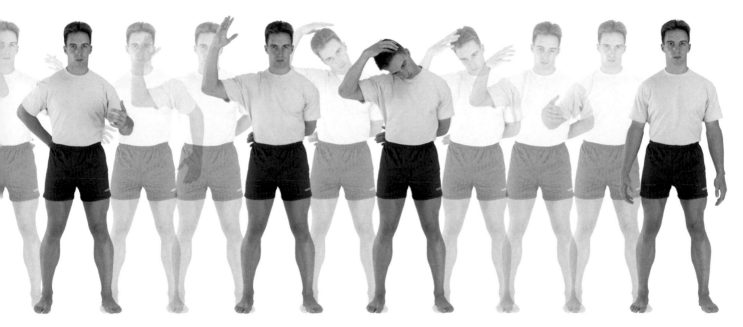

● Allow gravity to pull the head down so that it is leaning slightly forward and in line with the collar bone. Continue to stretch the neck by gently pulling downward and forward with your right arm.

● Your supporting arm will keep the left shoulder down, ensuring a more effective stretch. For safety, do not pull or push the head suddenly or move it into a position that is uncomfortable.

● Release the head, switch over hands and repeat the process on the other side, remembering to keep your neck relaxed throughout. Make sure that you keep your back straight and your legs soft at the knees.

● Now release the stretch and bring both arms to rest at your sides. Maintain a straight back, keep your knees soft, relax, and breathe deeply.

exhale ▶ begin to inhale ▶ inhale ‖ exhale ■

pre-exercise routine

standing hamstring, upper back and chest stretch

This is a progressive movement in two parts that will stretch your hamstrings, upper back, and chest muscles. This exercise does not need to be performed more than once. Hold the stretches for 20 seconds to gain the maximum benefit.

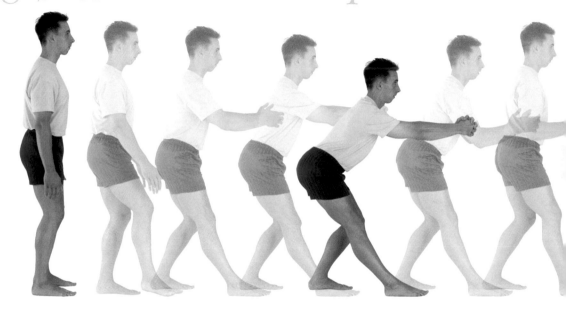

● Stand upright with your hands resting at your sides and your legs relaxed and slightly soft at the knees. Bring your right leg forward and place it roughly 22 inches (50 centimeters) in front of the other foot.

● Bend forward, flexing from the waist. At the same time, straighten your right leg to lock at the knee. The rear leg should remain soft and bent at the knee. Your hips should be square with both feet pointed forward and flat on the floor.

● Now extend your arms and raise them to chest height, interlacing your fingers to link your hands together. At the same time, continue to bend forward, pushing your buttocks out to create an arch in the back.

● Reach your arms out as far they will go, keeping your foot flat on the floor. You will feel a stretch in the hamstring muscles of your right leg and in the rhomboid muscles of your upper back. Hold the pose briefly.

inhale ▶ exhale ▶ ‖

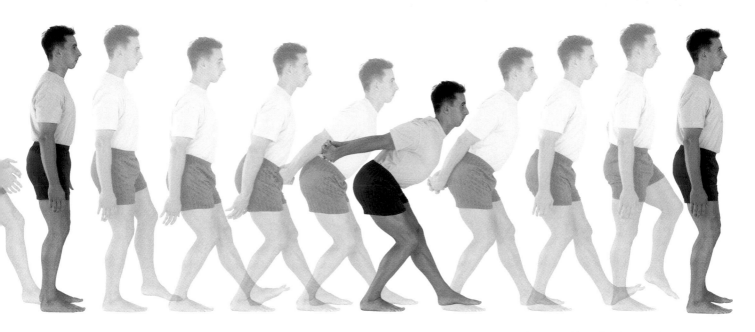

● Release the stretch, unclench your hands, and bring your arms back to your sides. Step your right foot back to align with the other foot and stand upright in preparation for the second part of the movement.

● Now step your left foot roughly 22 inches (50 centimeters) in front of the other foot. Bend forward, flexing from the waist. At the same time, straighten your right leg to lock at the knee. The rear leg should remain soft and bent at the knee.

● Bring both arms behind your back and link the fingers together to clench the hands. Extend the arms back and lock at the elbows while bending forward and pushing your buttocks out to arch your back. Keep your head up and push your chest out.

● You will feel a stretch across your chest and in the hamstring muscles of your left leg. Hold it briefly, before releasing the stretch. Now return to the standing upright position with your arms relaxed at your sides.

inhale ▶ begin to exhale ▶ exhale ‖ inhale ■

standing triceps and hips stretch

This is a progressive movement that will stretch the triceps, calves, and hip flexors. This exercise does not need to be performed more than once. Hold the stretch for at least 20 seconds to gain the maximum benefit.

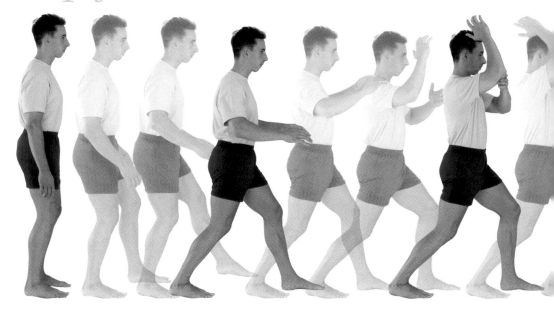

● Stand upright and facing forward with your hands resting at your sides and your legs relaxed and slightly soft at the knees.

● Slowly step your left leg forward and place it roughly 22 inches (50 centimeters) in front of the other foot, while at the same time raising both hands up in front of you.

● Raise your right arm and bring the hand and forearm behind your head so that the elbow is at 90 degrees. Bring your left hand up and over the top of your head to pull the right elbow to point vertically.

● Simultaneously, push your hips forward to create a gentle pull in your right hamstring and calf muscles. Do not allow the hips to rotate and keep your body weight centered.

| ■ | **begin to inhale** | ▶ | **inhale** | ▶ | **exhale** | ▶ |

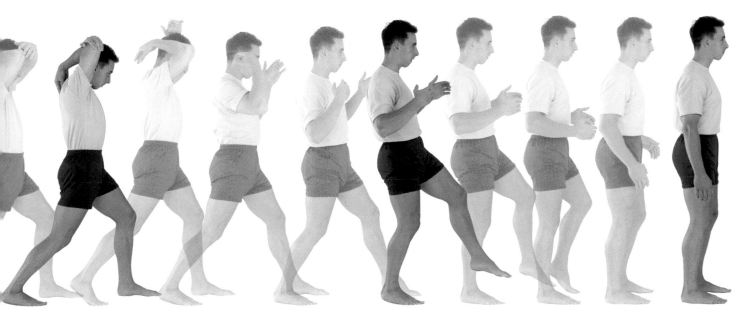

● Hold your elbow against your head with your hand resting downward between your shoulder blades. You will feel a stretch along your right triceps. Pulse the stretch for 20 seconds, pressing with the resting arm to maintain the pressure.

● At the same time, extend the stretch in the calves by shuffling the right leg backward while tilting the hips backward to stretch the hip flexors. To avoid arching your back, allow the upper body to lean forward slightly.

● Now release the stretch in your arms and bring them down to your sides. Lift your left leg and step it back to align with your right leg. Relax and inhale, pushing your chest out.

● Repeat the stretch on the other side, stepping your right leg forward and stretching the triceps in your left arm. Remember to keep your hips square and your body weight centered throughout the movement.

❚❚   inhale   ▶   exhale   ▶   ■

standing quadriceps and adductor stretch

This routine consists of two parts that works the quadriceps muscles in the front of the thigh and the adductor muscles on the insides of the thighs. Approach the quadriceps stretch with caution if you suffer from problems with your knees.

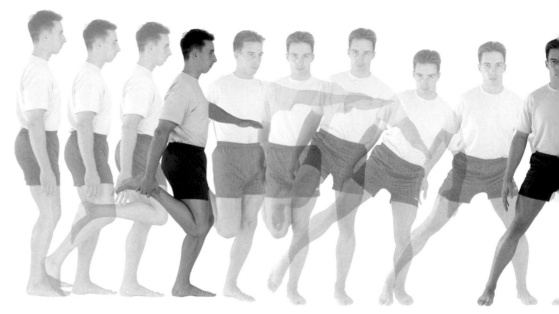

● Stand upright with your feet roughly three inches (eight centimeters) apart, your legs soft at the knees, and your arms resting at your sides.

● Bring your right foot up toward your buttocks, flexing at the knee. Hold the ankle of the raised foot with your right hand. Keep both thighs in line and hold your left arm out to help you balance on your standing leg.

● Keep your left leg soft at the knee for greater flexibility and balance and keep your hips pushed forward. Hold the leg for 20 seconds, pulling the leg higher to pulse the stretch. You will feel a stretch in your right quadriceps.

● Now release the foot and take your right leg out wide. Plant both feet firmly on the floor, roughly 36 inches (90 centimeters) apart with your toes pointing forward. Make sure your weight is evenly balanced across both legs.

begin to inhale ▶ **inhale** ❙❙ **begin to exhale** ▶

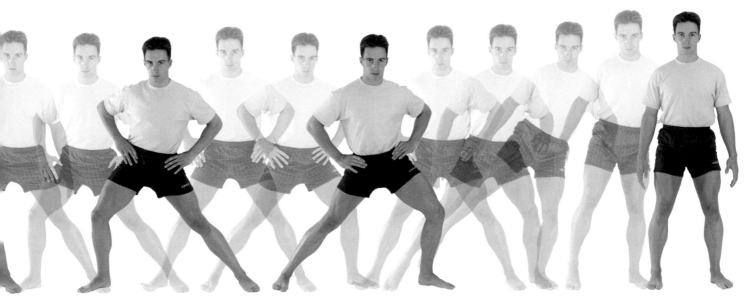

● Bring your hands up to rest on your hips and twist your body to the right side, bending your right knee. Raise the heel of your outstretched right leg off the floor. Do not let your bended knee protrude beyond the tips of your toes.

● Shuffle the outstretched left leg backward to find the stretch. You will feel a pull along the inside of the left thigh. Pulse the stretch for 20 seconds, rocking the hips down toward the outstretched leg for a full extension.

● Now bring your right knee in to stand with your feet spaced evenly and your body weight centered. Repeat the stretch on the other side, bending your right knee and stretching your left leg. Keep your hands on your hips throughout the movement.

● Release the stretch and bring both legs in to stand upright and soft at the knees, with your spine straight and your hands relaxed at your sides.

exhale   ‖   begin to inhale   ▶   inhale   ‖   ◼

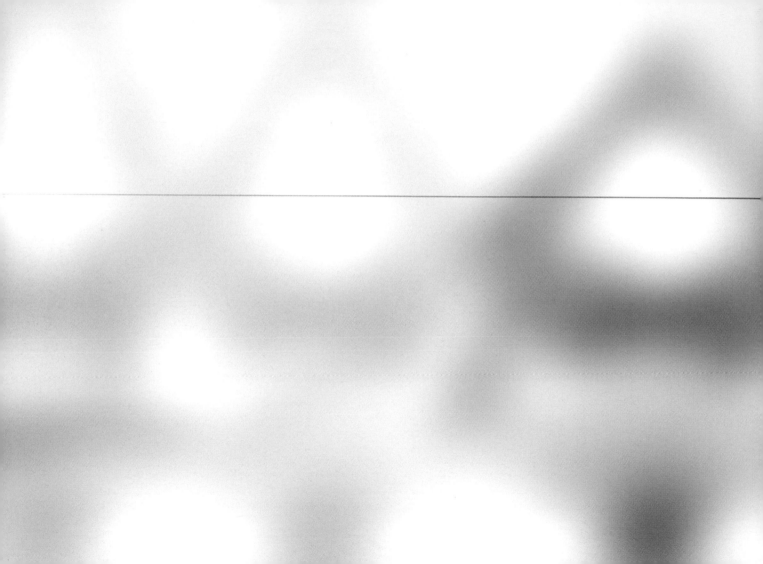

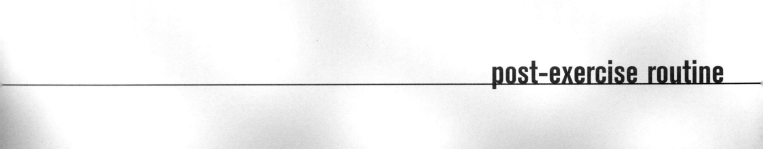

seated hamstring stretch

This is a simple routine for stretching the hamstring muscles at the back of the thighs. For safety, do not hold the stretch if you feel any discomfort in your lower back.

● To begin this exercise, sit upright with your back straight, your legs extended, and your arms at your sides with the palms resting flat on the floor.

● Raise your right leg and take the knee out sideways so that it is bent at 90 degrees. Rest the sole of your foot against the inside of your outstretched leg, just below the knee. For comfort, you can use a rolled towel to support the ankle of your extended leg.

● Bending from the waist, lean forward and reach your hands toward your extended foot. Grasp the foot with both hands, keeping your head facing forward.

● Pull against the sole of your foot. You will feel a stretch in the hamstrings of your left leg. Pulse the stretch for 10 seconds. Keep the toes pointed forward to ensure the stretch is in the thigh; otherwise, the pull will stay in the shin.

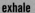

■   inhale   ▶   exhale   ▶   inhale   **11**

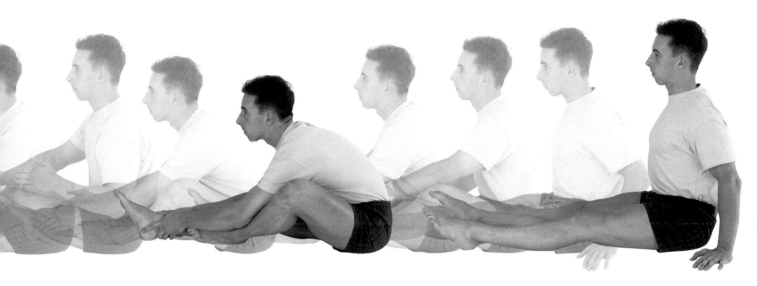

● Release the stretch, withdraw your hands from your foot, and sit upright. Now extend your right leg flat on the floor. Bring your left leg out, bent at the knee to 90 degrees, to rest the sole of the foot against the inside of your right leg.

● Bend forward and perform the stretch on the other side. Remember to keep the toes pointed forward to ensure the stretch is in the thigh, otherwise, the pull will stay in the shin.

● Pulse the stretch for 10 seconds. You will feel a stretch in the hamstrings of your right leg. (If you have difficulty reaching the sole of your foot, bend the extended leg slightly to bring the foot closer.)

● Now raise your head, straighten your back, and extend your left leg in line with the right leg. Place your hands at your sides and relax.

exhale   inhale   ❚❚   exhale   inhale   ▶   exhale   ■

lying quadriceps and hips stretch *flexors*

This exercise stretches the quadriceps (the muscles at the front of the thighs) and the hips through knee flexion. If you suffer from weak knees, do not pull the joint too tightly.

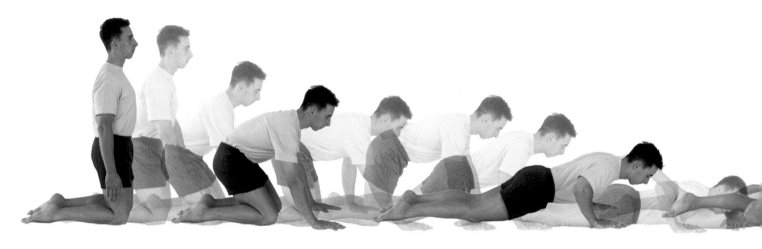

● To begin the move, kneel with your body upright and facing forward. Slowly lower your upper body toward the floor.

● Kneel on all fours, with your palms pressed flat on the floor and your arms roughly shoulder width apart. Ease your body weight forward onto your arms and shoulders.

● Continue to ease your upper body forward, taking the weight with your arms while keeping your shins and feet flat on the floor. Keeping your back straight throughout the movement, lower yourself to rest flat on the floor.

● Lying flat, bring your left arm to the front and relax your head on your forearm. To begin the stretch, flex your right leg at the knee and bring the foot toward your buttocks, meeting the ankle with your right hand.

■   **inhale**   **exhale**   ▶   **inhale**   ▶   **exhale**   ▶

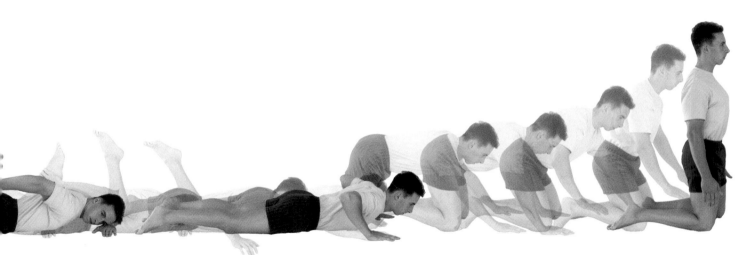

● Grip your ankle and pull the leg back into the body, so that the heel is roughly three inches (eight centimeters) from the buttocks. Push the hip into the floor to lift the knee from the ground to increase the stretch.

● You will feel a stretch in your quadriceps and along the outside of your right hip. Hold the position for a few breaths. Now release the leg. Extend your leg back toward the floor so that it is lying flat.

● Using both arms, push the body upward into a kneeling position (as though you are doing push-ups). Continue to push upward, keeping your knees on the floor, until you are again resting on all fours.

● Keep your back straight, taking care not to arch it throughout the movement. Lift your body back into the kneeling, upright position and let your arms relax at your sides.

‖   **inhale**   ▶   **exhale**   ▶   **breathe normally**   ■

hips and back extension

This simple exercise will stretch your spine, chest, and abdomen. Once your have become familiar with the basic pose, you can exaggerate the movement to achieve an even greater stretch.

● Kneel on the floor, with your body upright, your spine straight, and your head facing forward. Keep your arms relaxed at your sides.

● Now slowly lower your hips toward your heels, flexing at the knees. Bring your buttocks down so that they are approximately three inches (eight centimeters) from the back of your feet; any closer could cause the knee joints to compress.

● At the same time, bring your hands back toward your feet while resting your outstretched fingers on the floor with your arms extended. Use your arms to take the weight and guide the body back by walking your hands along the floor.

● Continue to lower your body backward so that your palms rest flat on the floor and your arms are fully extended and locked at the elbows.

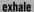

| | inhale | ▶ | exhale | ▶ | inhale | ▶ |

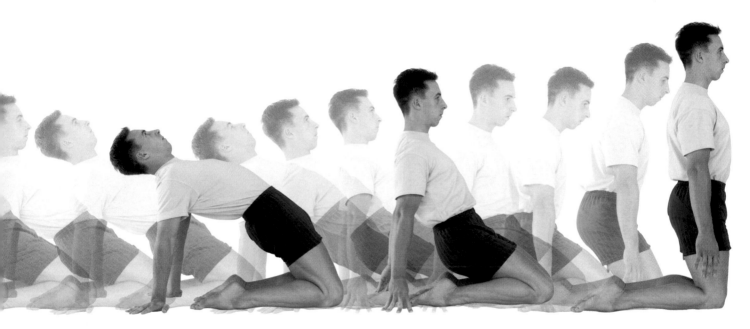

● Bearing your body weight on your arms, push your hips and chest upward and bring your head back to face the sky. Keep the head in line with the spine. Keep your elbows locked.

● Hold the stretch for 10 seconds, or for as long as it feels comfortable. You will feel a stretch in your hips, abdomen, and chest, and along the length of the spine. To extend the stretch, exaggerate the movement by pushing the hips forward.

● Release the stretch, first bringing your hips back down to just above your heels. Extend your fingers to take the body weight as you raise yourself into an upright position.

● Flexing at the knees, lift your upper body to kneel upright. Bring your arms back to your sides. Face forward with your spine straight and relax.

exhale   ‖   inhale   ▶   exhale   ▶   **breathe normally**   ■

lying adductor wall stretch

This exercise is a progressive movement that will stretch the adductor muscles on the insides of the thighs. You will need to lie with your feet up against a wall to perform this stretch effectively.

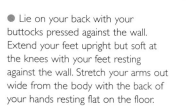

● Lie on your back with your buttocks pressed against the wall. Extend your feet upright but soft at the knees with your feet resting against the wall. Stretch your arms out wide from the body with the back of your hands resting flat on the floor.

● Slowly slide your legs down the wall toward your body, bringing your knees out wide and the soles of your feet together. Take your knees out to an angle of 90 degrees.

● Bring your hands up to rest on your knees, then gently push your knees into the wall, keeping them aligned and even throughout the movement. Gravity will provide resistance. You will feel a progressive stretch along the insides of your thighs.

● Give a strong push with your hands. At the furthest push, open the legs and allow them to drop away from each other. Part your feet and rest your hands above your knees to press down on the legs to extend the stretch.

■   **inhale**   ▶   **exhale**   ❚❚   **inhale**   ▶

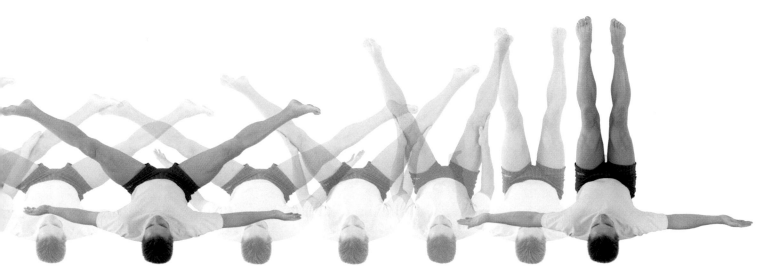

● Now slowly extend your legs until they are fully stretched apart to form a 90 degree angle from the center. Bring your hands up to hold the insides of your knee joints to provide support. You will feel a stretch in the gracilis muscle in the inner thigh.

● Hold the stretch briefly, then progress the move by bringing your hands away from the legs and extending your arms out to the sides. Let gravity take the legs down as far as they will go to achieve a full stretch.

● Now release the stretch and bring your legs back together, using your hands to guide and support them into position. Keep your heels against the wall throughout to maintain balance.

● Bring both feet back together so that they are roughly three inches (eight centimeters) apart, with your legs soft at the knees. Bring your arms out wide from the center to rest on the floor in the starting position.

exhale   ‖   **inhale**   ▶   **exhale**   ▶   ‖

seated gluteal stretch *lower back*

This exercise comes in two parts and will stretch the gluteal and lower back muscles. Be careful not to pull the leg too tightly into the body if you have a lower back or gluteal injury.

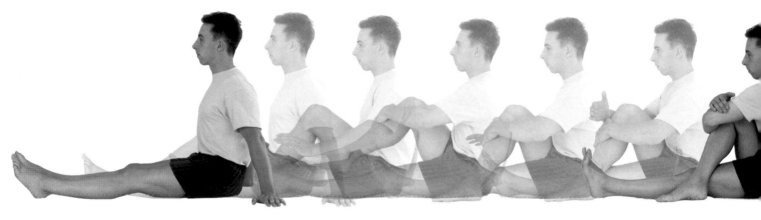

● Sit upright, with both legs extended forward and flat on the floor. Now slowly bring your right foot in toward your body, raising your knee into an upright position as you do so.

● Bring your foot back so that it is level with the knee of the opposite leg. Now use your hands to guide the foot over the opposite knee and rest the sole of the foot on the floor, parallel to and resting against the opposite knee.

● Wrap both arms around the knee and hug it in toward the chest. Let the knee slot into the angle of the inside of the elbow joint for comfort. The heel of the raised leg should stay on the floor throughout the stretch.

● Hold the position and feel a stretch in the gluteal muscles of your right thigh and buttocks. Make sure that the ankle aligns comfortably with the knee to avoid any unpleasant twists as you maintain an upright posture.

■   **inhale**   ▶   **exhale**   ▶   **inhale**   ❚❚

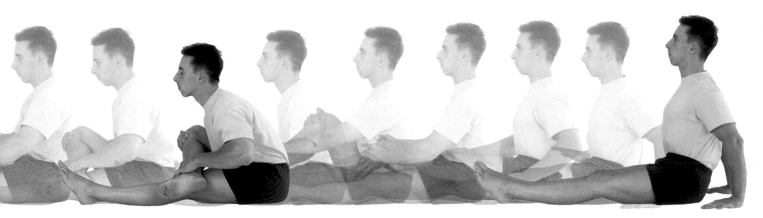

● Release the hug and lower your knee to the right. Simultaneously, lift the right foot from the floor and rest your right ankle on the opposite thigh, holding the ankle in close to the body. The right shin should now be 90 degrees to the opposite leg.

● Gently lean forward, while holding your right ankle with your left hand and your knee with your right hand. You will feel a stretch in the upper part of your buttocks and your lower back. Hold the position briefly. Keep your head up throughout the stretch.

● Release the stretch and gently raise your back to an upright position. Guide your right leg out and away from your body with your hands. Extend your right leg to rest flat on the floor in the sitting posture. Relax both legs and breathe deeply.

● Bring your arms behind your back and rest the hands flat on the floor for support. Now repeat both stretches using the other leg.

exhale ▶ inhale ❚❚ exhale ▶ inhale ▶ exhale ◼

lower back mobilization *and hips*

The lying down twist is a popular yoga position that will stretch your lower back muscles, increase spinal mobility, and open up the chest. This routine is one of the best ways of realigning the spinal fluid and should be performed after any back stretching movements.

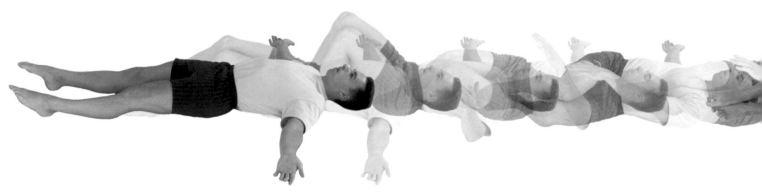

● Do not perform this exercise if you have recently suffered a lower back injury. Lie on your back with your arms extended by your sides and at 90 degrees to the body. Slowly raise your legs, bringing your knees together.

● Bring your knees up to make a 90 degree angle at the joint. Raise your hands and bring them toward your knees, keeping your back, shoulders, and head flat on the floor.

● Keeping your knees together, gently push your right knee with your left hand down toward the floor. Pull the knees downward and flat against the floor, using your left hand to apply pressure on the thigh.

● Stretch your resting arm along the floor and away from the body. This will provide support and ensure that your shoulders remain firmly pressed down. It is important to keep your shoulders pressed flat on the floor to achieve the correct stretch.

■ inhale   exhale ▶   inhale ▶   exhale ▶

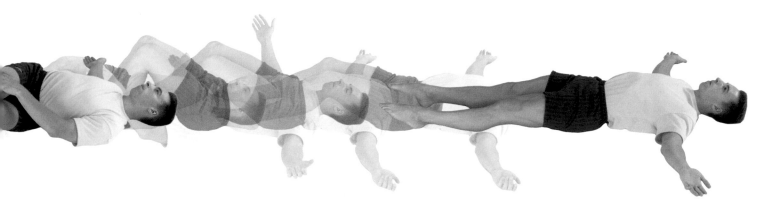

● Hold the pose for three breaths, pressing the knees to the floor with your left hand, and keeping your head facing upward. You will feel your spine loosen and a stretch along the outside of your thigh.

● Release the stretch and raise your knees to the upright position with the soles of your feet flat on the floor. Bring your hands back to your sides.

● Now lower your legs and stretch them out so that they are again flat against the floor. Open your arms outward and rest them against the floor with palms facing upward.

● Now repeat the stretch on the other side, remembering to keep your shoulders level and against the floor.

inhale   II   exhale   ▶   inhale   ▶   exhale   ■

seated calf, chest and back stretch

This exercise consists of two counterposed movements that will stretch your calves and lower back.

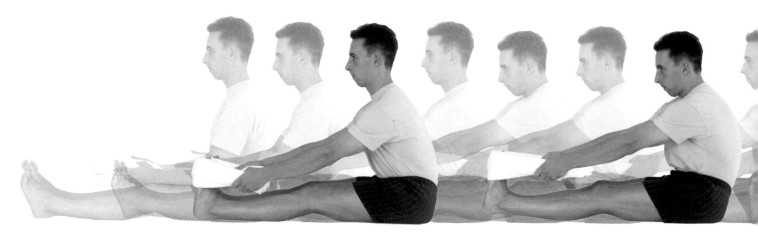

● Sit upright on the floor with your back straight, legs outstretched, ankles close together, and the soles of your feet facing outward.

● Hook the towel around the upper part of the soles of both feet. Hold the towel with both hands in such a way that you have to lean forward to take up the tension. Keep your calves pressed flat against the floor.

● Gently pull on the towel so that your feet lift from the ground by one or up to an inch (two centimeters). You will feel a stretch in your calves. Pull with your arms and hold the pose briefly.

● Continue the stretch by pulling from the back, pushing your shoulders forward and rounding your back. This will allow you to stretch your upper back muscles. Now release the stretch by relaxing your arms and releasing the towel.

inhale ▶ **exhale** ‖ **inhale** ‖ **exhale**

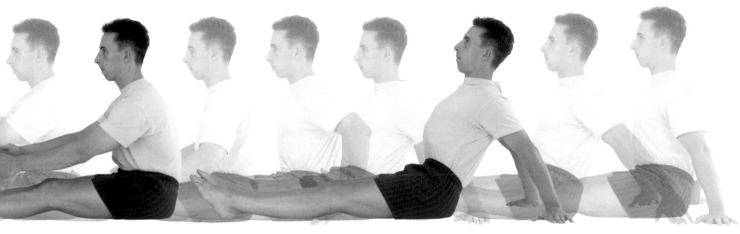

● Now bring your arms back and away from your feet and slowly straighten your back. Flexing from the waist, gradually lean backward, taking your arms behind you as you do so.

● Extend your arms and rest the palms of your hands flat on the floor, approximately 12 inches (25 centimeters) away from your buttocks. For safety, make sure your hands are pointing at 90 degrees from the body.

● Lean backward, pushing your chest out and keeping your abdomen tight. As you lean back you will feel a stretch in your chest and spine, and a light stretch in your shoulders.

● Now release the stretch and bring your hands forward to rest on the floor in line with your buttocks. Relax and breathe deeply.

inhale ▶ **exhale** ▶ **inhale** ‖ **exhale** ▶ ■

kneeling triceps, lats and deltoid stretch *and deltoids*

This routine stretches the latissimus dorsi, triceps, and posterior deltoids in a progressive movement. The kneeling stance is effective because it forces the quadriceps to stretch to balance the body throughout the routine.

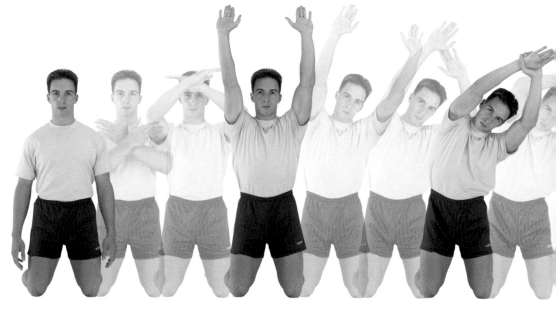

● Begin this routine kneeling on the floor with your arms relaxed at your sides. Your knees should be spaced approximately shoulder width apart and planted firmly on the floor.

● Now slowly raise your hands to cross your wrists in front of your chest, before opening the arms out as you reach your hands upward toward the sky. This opening out movement will help your breathing.

● With your arms fully outstretched and your palms facing outward, slowly bend your body to the left, flexing from the waist. Bring your left hand over to grasp the wrist of your right arm and pull the arm out and away from the body.

● You will feel a stretch along the right side of your body in the latissimus dorsi muscles. Progress the stretch by pulsing the movement.

inhale ▶ **exhale** ▶ **inhale** ❙❙ **exhale**

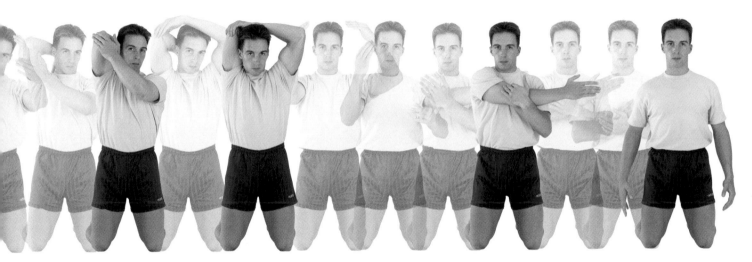

● To begin the triceps stretch, release the hand and move your right arm behind your head so that the hand is resting between your shoulder blades. Bring your left hand up to press your elbow back to point vertically.

● Hold your elbow against your head with your hand resting downward between your shoulder blades. You will feel a stretch along your right triceps. Pulse the stretch for 20 seconds, pressing with the resting arm to maintain the pressure.

● Release the stretch and bring your right arm down. Reach your right arm across your chest, fully extended with the hand pointing to the right and parallel with the left shoulder. Hug your right arm into the body, pressing the upper arm with your left hand.

● You will feel a stretch in your posterior deltoid. Release the stretch and lower your arms to relax at your sides. Now perform the exercise on the other side, stretching your left triceps and latissimus dorsi.

inhale   ▶   exhale   ❚❚   inhale   ❚❚   exhale   ■

back stretches

seated back and neck stretch

This is a mild, progressive stretch that will exercise the muscles of the back (the erector spinae) and neck. It is a good movement for those who have an excessively curved lower spine, as it stretches and extends the muscles in this area.

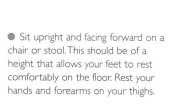
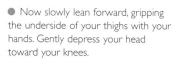
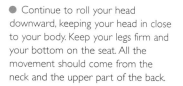

● Sit upright and facing forward on a chair or stool. This should be of a height that allows your feet to rest comfortably on the floor. Rest your hands and forearms on your thighs.

● Now slowly lean forward, gripping the underside of your thighs with your hands. Gently depress your head toward your knees.

● Continue to roll your head downward, keeping your head in close to your body. Keep your legs firm and your bottom on the seat. All the movement should come from the neck and the upper part of the back.

● Your back will curve slightly. Continue the downward movement until you feel a stretch along the length of your back. Hold the stretch, breathing as deeply as possible.

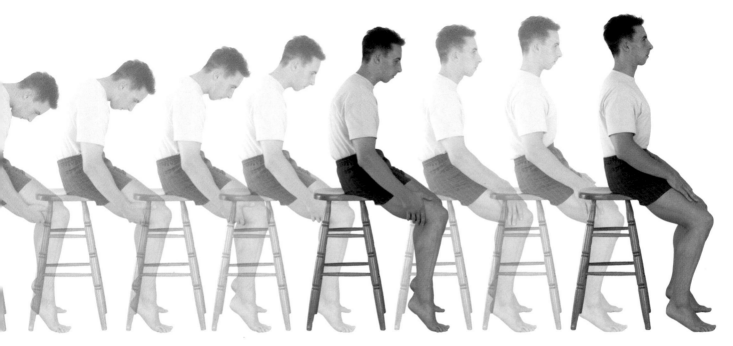

● If you feel a pull in your stomach muscles as you depress your body, release the stretch to a more comfortable position.

● Now exhale and release the stretch. Come out of the position by gradually raising your head and pulling your back up straight.

● Bring your hands from under your thighs and rest them again on the top of your thighs. Face forward, straighten your back, and lift your head upright in one flowing movement.

● You can perform this stretch a number of times to work the lower back and massage the spine.

▶ **inhale**　　　▶　　　**exhale**　　　▶　　　■

hamstrings with stool

This is a progressive
movement that will stretch
your hamstring muscles.
You will need a low stool or
step and a rolled-up towel
to perform this movement
effectively.

● Place your right foot on a low stool with the ankle rested on a towel so that the foot is raised to roughly the same height as the knee of the standing leg. Shuffle your standing leg back so that the raised leg is roughly 60 degrees from the standing leg.

● If you suffer from knee problems, keep your extended leg slightly bent throughout the stretch.

● To begin the stretch, raise your hands and bring them to rest on top of your extended thigh, just above the knee, with the fingers pointing along the length of the leg toward the foot.

● Now slowly lean your upper body forward, bending from the waist, and keeping your back straight. Keep your standing leg soft throughout the forward bend so that it bears your body weight.

▶   **inhale**   ▶   **exhale**   ▶

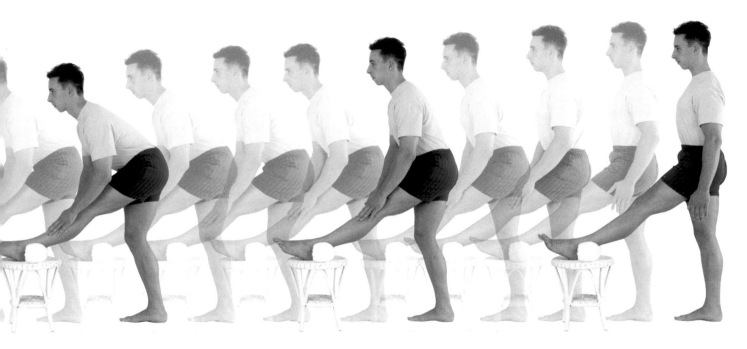

● Continue to lean forward, bringing your body lower, while sliding your hands down your leg. Keep your elbows bent and your head up throughout the stretch.

● You will feel a progressive stretch down the hamstring muscles on the back of your left thigh. At the furthest reach, your hands should be resting on the upper part of the shin.

● Once your body weight has tipped forward and on to your outstretched leg, you should reverse the move. Raise your body, moving your hands back up your leg in a slow movement.

● Bring your head and upper body into an upright position and bring your hands to your sides to relax. Now perform the stretch with the other leg, remembering to keep your body weight on your standing leg.

‖   inhale   ▶   exhale   ▶   ‖

standing knee flexor *calves and hip flexors*

This gentle, progressive exercise will stretch your calves and hip flexors. The movement is split into an easy and an advanced stretch. By performing them in turn, you can avoid putting your muscles under unnecessary strain.

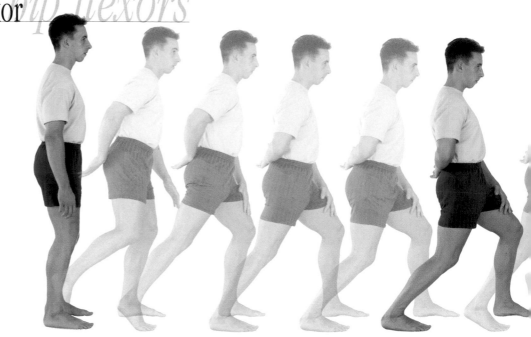

● Stand upright, with your feet slightly apart, your knees soft, and your arms relaxed at your sides.

● Place your right forearm behind your back, resting in the small of your back for support. Take your right leg 24 inches (50 centimeters) backward and place your foot flat on the floor. Do not step back too far, as this can rotate the hips.

● Bend the front knee and rest your left hand on your extended left thigh. Lean backward, simultaneously bringing your torso up straight and pushing your hips forward.

● Keep your hips square and your back straight throughout the movement. Try to avoid arching your back by keeping your upper body upright. Now push against the front leg to extend the stretch. Hold the pose and pulse the stretch.

■　　　　　　　**inhale**　▶　　　　　　　　　▶　　　　　**exhale**　❚❚　　　▶

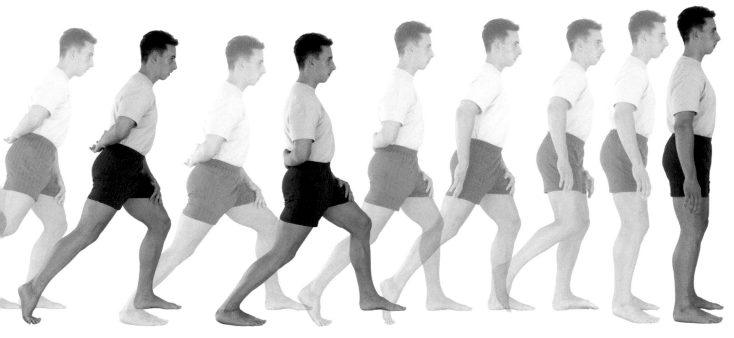

● Now release the stretch, bring your body upright, and shuffle your right leg backward. Extend the stretch further. Hold the pose and pulse the stretch, keeping your hips forward.

● Repeat the process as far as it feels comfortable to do so, remembering not to let your back arch.

● Now release the pose and step your right leg forward. Bring your arms back to your sides and relax in the standing upright position.

● Repeat the movement with the other leg, practicing both easy and advanced stretches in turn.

| inhale | ▶ | exhale | ‖ | breathe normally | ▶ | ■ |

spine

mobilization of the back

This movement is in two parts and arches the back upward and inward. It will mobilize the spine and ensure that the spinal fluid is restored to its original position after lower back stretches. Keep the movement slow and relaxed and repeat it two or three times to gain the full benefit.

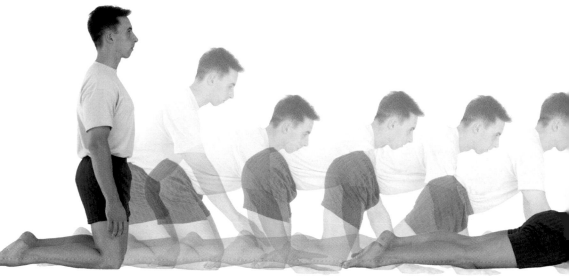

● Begin the exercise kneeling on the floor with your body upright and your arms relaxed at your sides. Your knees should be close together but not touching, with your feet pointing away from your body.

● Now lean forward, bending from the waist, and bring your arms down to rest the palms flat on the floor. Keep your back straight throughout the forward bend.

● Walk your hands forward and continue to extend your body. Lower your hips to the ground while keeping your upper body raised with the palms of your hands.

● Let the lower body sink to create an inverse arch in the back. Keep your head up and face forward. Hold the pose briefly, pulsing the stretch by pressing down with the palms.

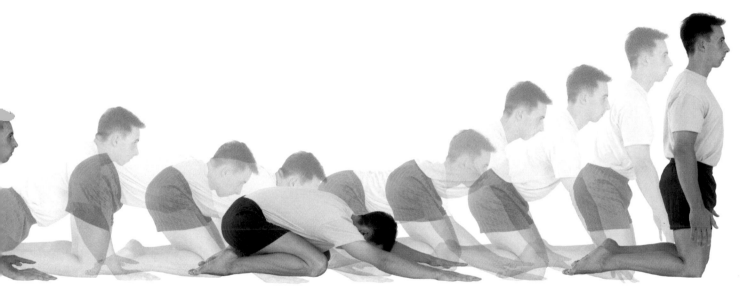

● Release the pose and lift yourself off the floor and back on to your hands and knees, with your back straight and hips aligned.

● Now lower your buttocks backward toward your feet and bring your chest down to rest on your thighs. Keep your hands flat on the floor throughout the movement. Bring your head down to face the floor.

● Push back on your haunches so that your arms are fully extended with palms flat on the floor. Hold the pose for 20 seconds to gain an upward arch of the back. Do not press your buttocks back on to your feet, as this can compress the knee joints.

● Now release the stretch and lift the hips to bring the body into an upright position. Keep your back straight throughout the movement. Kneel fully upright, facing forward, and relax your arms at your sides.

▶   **inhale**   **exhale**   ‖   ▶   **inhale**   **exhale**   ■

cat *abdominal and spinal flexibility*

This well-known yoga posture includes two counterposes to arch the back both upward and downward. This movement will mobilize the spinal fluid, improve spinal flexibility, and stretch the back muscles and abdomen.

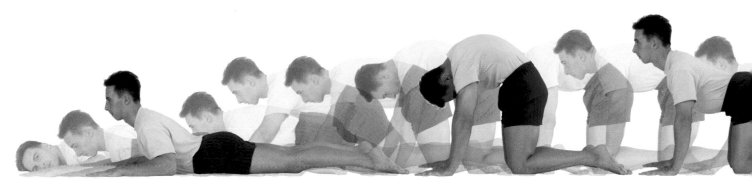

● Lie flat with your legs outstretched and your forearms and the palms of your hands flat against the floor with your elbows out at the sides. Your head should be rested on the floor between your hands.

● Now slowly raise your head and push against the floor with your hands to lift your chest from the floor. Flexing at the knees, lift your hips from the floor to bring yourself up on to all fours with your arms locked at the elbows. Face down toward the floor.

● All your weight should now be on your hands and knees. Walk your hands backward a few inches to arch your back upward in the Cat pose. Hold the pose and pulse the stretch by bending your head inward.

● Now release the stretch and lift your head up while simultaneously pushing your buttocks outward. Push your chest down to gain an inverted arch in the back. Hold the pose. You will feel a stretch in your lower back.

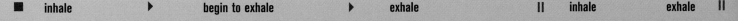

■ inhale   ▶   begin to exhale   ▶   exhale   ‖   inhale   exhale   ‖

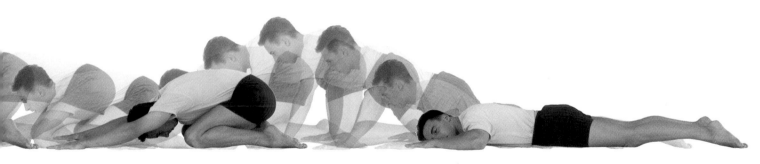

● Release the stretch and lower your buttocks down toward your feet. Bring your chest forward to rest on your thighs and your head down to face the floor. Keep your hands flat on the floor throughout the movement.

● Push back on your haunches so that your arms are fully extended with palms flat on the floor. Hold the pose for 20 seconds and stretch the spine. Do not press your buttocks back on to your feet, as this can compress the knee joints.

● Release the stretch and lift your body, bringing your hips up so that you rest on all fours. Extending from the knee joint, continue the forward movement to bring your chest back down on to the floor.

● Extend your legs fully, lie your head on the floor, and rest your hands besides your head with your elbows at 90 degrees. Relax and breathe deeply.

▶ **inhale**   **exhale**   ❙❙   **inhale**   ▶   **exhale**   ■

rotated gluteal stretch *lower back*

This is a progressive
movement that will stretch the
gluteal muscles and gently
stretch and twist the spine.
When twisting the body,
remember to support yourself
on at least one arm to avoid
damaging your spine.

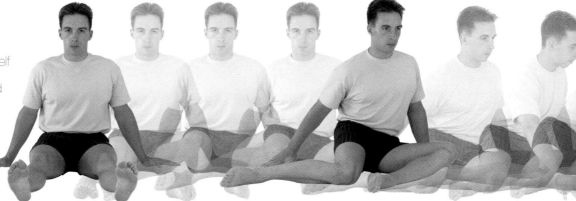

● Sit on the floor with your legs
extended and your feet roughly
shoulder width apart. Rest the palms
of your hands flat on the floor to
support your back.

● Begin the move by bringing both
legs into your left side, drawing the
knees in toward the body. Support
your body with your arms while
performing this move. The sides of
your legs should now be lying flat on
the floor.

● Now rotate your body to the left,
twisting from the waist. To avoid
compressing the knee joints, do not
bend the knees beyond 90 degrees.

● Now move the hands around to
the left side of the hips and begin to
lean forward, using your arms to take
your weight as your bend. For safety,
transfer your arms one at a time so
that the spine is always supported.

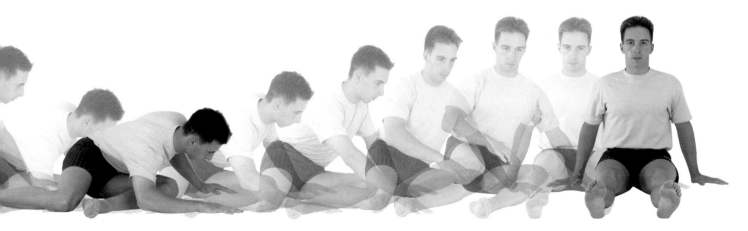

● With the palms of your hands flat on the floor, lower your chest downward. Try to keep the back straight and do not slouch when leaning forward.

● Hold the pose briefly. You will feel a stretch in the spine. Now bring yourself away from the floor, performing the movement in reverse.

● Bring your legs out from under your body, remembering to keep at least one hand on the floor to ensure that your back is supported throughout the twisting movement. Bring your hips back to face forward.

● Return to the start position with your legs extended and your arms locked at the elbow with palms resting flat at your sides. Now repeat the exercise on the other side.

II   ▶   **inhale**   ▶   ▶   **exhale**   ■

dynamic stretches

standing rotation *dorsi, quadratus lumborum*

This exercise is a continuous flowing movement that stretches the latissimus dorsi and quadratus lumborum muscles. The latissimus dorsi extends and retracts the humerus (upper arm) in combination with the pectoralis muscle.

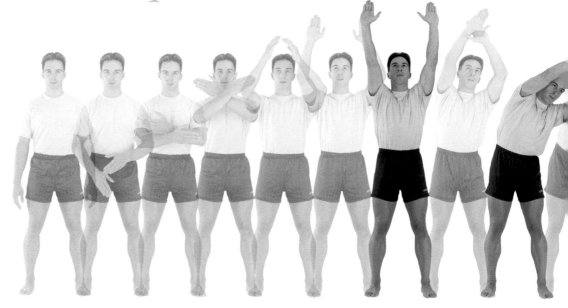

- Stand with your feet roughly shoulder width apart. Keep your legs soft at the knees. Inhale and slowly raise your arms and cross them in front of your chest.

- Continue to raise your hands and cross them at the wrists. Move the arms in an upward, expanding movement. You should be fully inhaled as your hands reach head height.

- Extend your hands toward the sky, facing your head upward as you do. Tilt your head upward and exhale as your hands reach skyward.

- Now start to lean to your left, flexing from the waist. Grasp your right hand with your left hand to help pull your body downward in a gradual rotation. Remember to keep your back straight.

inhale ▶ exhale ‖ inhale ‖

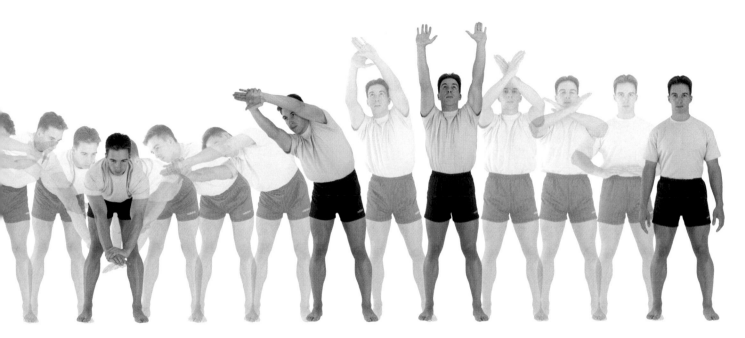

● Continue the downward rotation by pulling your right arm with your left hand. Gradually move into a forward rotation. At the lowest point, your back should be bent forward at 90 degrees. Let your shoulders drop and exhale.

● At the lowest point of the rotation you will feel a stretch in your hamstrings. Stick out your buttocks to ensure that your back remains straight. Do not let the body slouch. Switch hands to continue the movement.

● Reverse the movement to continue the rotation upward to your left, leading with your straight arm. Continue the stretch and reach both hands skyward to achieve a full stretch in the latissimus dorsi. Inhale as you reach upward.

● Lower the arms, pulling the hands downward, and bring them back to your sides. Relax your body.

exhale   ‖   inhale   ‖   exhale   ▶   breathe normally   ■

walking hamstrings *latissimus dorsi, rhomboids*

This is a progressive exercise that combines to stretch the hamstrings, the latissimus dorsi, and the rhomboid muscles on the shoulders.

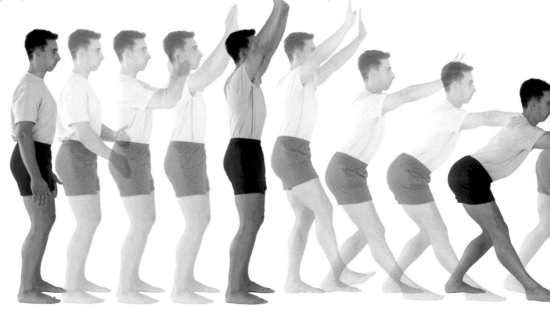

● For safety reasons, make sure that you reach forward and keep your hands beyond your head throughout the movement; a more vertical reach could result in back strain or injury.

● Stand upright, with your feet pointing forward and your legs soft at the knees. Slowly raise your arms and bring them across your chest. Inhale. Continue to reach your arms skyward, with palms facing outward.

● Exhale as your arms pass the crown of your head. Reach skyward as far as your can with palms facing upward. You will feel a stretch in your back. Now inhale and slowly slide your right foot forward while lowering your arms and reaching forward.

● Continue to reach forward, pushing your arms in front of you. Lower your back while keeping your spine straight. Keep your hips aligned and push your bottom out for balance.

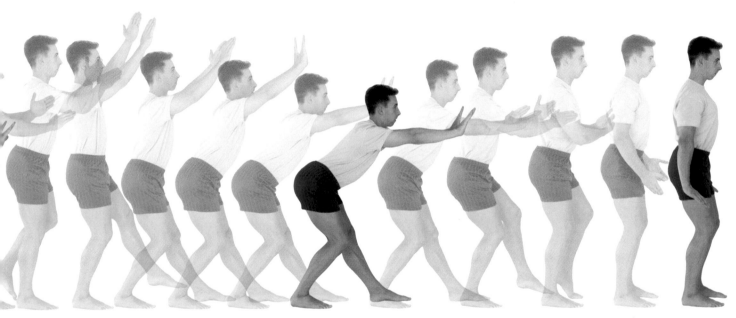

● Hold the pose and feel a stretch at the back of the neck, in the latissimus dorsi muscles and in the hamstrings. Your legs should remain aligned as far as the knee for stability and balance.

● Now gently raise your body, flexing from the waist, and step your left leg forward, keeping your arms raised throughout the movement.

● Step forward with the other leg and repeat the stretch on the other side. Exhale and reach upward, then inhale and reach forward with palms facing outward. Keep your back straight and legs stable at the lowest point of the reach.

● Hold the pose, then bring both feet forward, bring your arms down, and return to the standing upright position with arms relaxed at your sides.

exhale ▶ **inhale** ‖ **exhale** ▶ ‖

quadriceps stretch with abductor reaches

This sequence of movements combines quadriceps stretches on both legs with extended reaches and abductor stretches to both sides. It is also a good exercise for helping you to improve your balance.

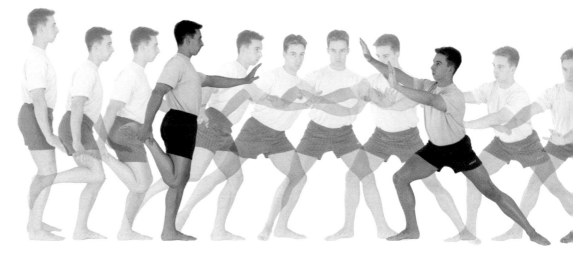

● Starting in the standing position, place your feet about 12 inches (30 centimeters) apart. Let your arms hang loosely at your sides and check that the knees are soft, not locked. Hold your shoulders back and your head upright and facing forward.

● Supporting the body weight on your left leg, raise your right leg up to the buttocks, flexing at the knee. Take your right hand back to meet the raised leg and grasp hold of the ankle.

● With your right hand, guide the heel to within two to three inches (six to eight centimeters) of the buttocks and hold the pose. At the same time, push your left arm forward to help maintain balance.

● Release the right foot and step it back, turning the body to the front. Push both arms out in front of you and rotate them to the right. Rotate your right foot to the right and bend the knee. You will feel a stretch in the oblique muscles on your left side.

■   **inhale**   ▶   **exhale**   ‖   **inhale**   ▶

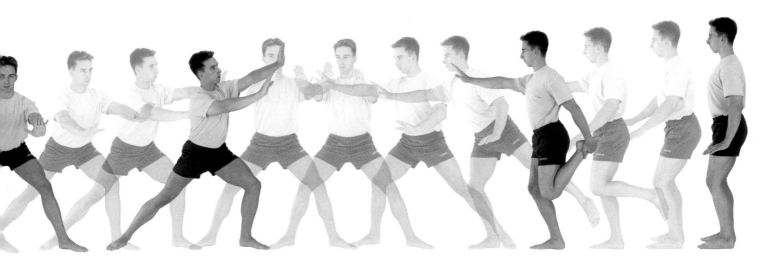

● Rotate to the front, keeping the feet at a 45 degree angle to allow good rotation. As you turn, make sure that the weight-bearing leg rotates to avoid damaging the knee. Check that your hips remain square.

● With both arms still outstretched, rotate to the left. Swivel your left foot to the side and flex the knee. Check that your head follows the direction and angle of your arms, to create a strong diagonal across the body.

● Rotate again to the right, letting the left hand fall back to the side. Raise your left leg and flex the knee. Grasp the foot with your left hand and hold it two to three inches (six to eight centimeters) away from the buttocks.

● Hold the stretch, using your outstretched right arm to help keep your balance. Release the left foot and lower your leg to the ground, to stand with your feet slightly apart. At the same time, lower your arms.

exhale ▶ inhale ❙❙ ▶ exhale ❙❙ ▶ ■

standing calf and hip flexor
gastrocnemius and illiacus psoas

This is a progressive movement that will stretch the calves and hips. The sequence consists of a right leg extension, with both arms extended; a right leg extension with one arm extended; and a left leg extension with both arms extended.

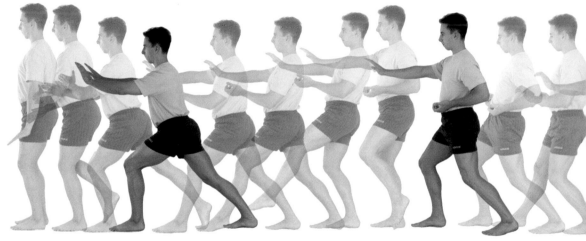

● Stand upright with your knees relaxed. Now slowly raise your right leg and step it backward, making sure that the other leg bears your weight.

● Press the heel of your right leg down toward the floor to gain a full extension. Simultaneously, raise your hands and push both arms forward as if pressing against a wall. Pushing with the arms will help you to stretch your heel flexor further.

● Keep your resting leg bent at the knee, but do not allow the knee joint to extend beyond the end of your left toes. For correct posture, keep your hips square, chest forward, and head up throughout the movement.

● Now lift your left leg and take a step backward, withdrawing your left arm as you do so, but keeping your right arm outstretched. Now push your hips forward as you take your arms back.

■   **inhale**   **||**   **exhale**   ▶   **inhale**   **||**

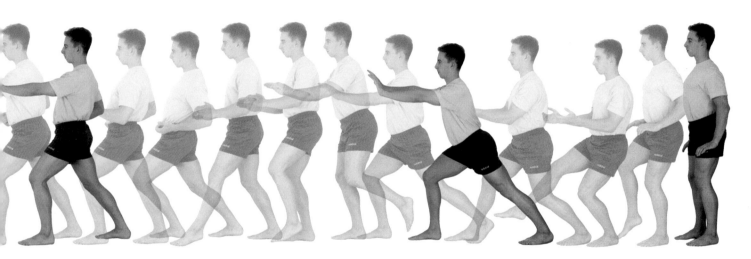

● Continue the backward movement and step back your right leg. Simultaneously lower your right arm and extend your left arm. Remember to keep your hips square and your chest out throughout the movement.

● Continue the movement and step your left leg backward. Shift your weight to your right leg and extend your left leg backward. Again, push your hips forward and bring your arms backward.

● As you fully extend your left leg backward, again push out both arms as though pressing against a wall. Keep your resting leg bent at the knee and do not let your knee joint extend beyond the ends of your toes.

● Return to the standing upright position. Finish the exercise with your knees relaxed and your hands resting at your sides.

exhale   ‖   inhale   ▶   exhale   ‖   ▶   ■

cross-legged gluteal stretch

gluteals and lower back

This exercise stretches the gluteal muscles by isolating them through sitting cross legged on the floor. The lean forward will stretch the gluteus maximus muscles, while the rotation will cover all the major muscle groups.

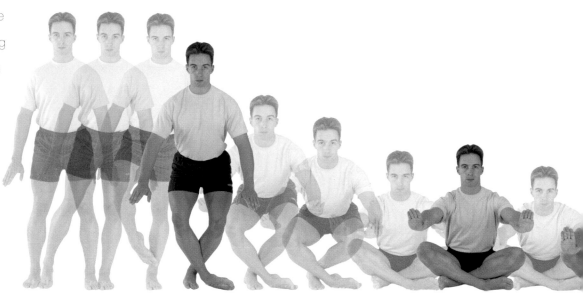

● Begin by standing with your feet shoulder width apart and your hands loose at your sides.

● Slowly cross your legs and lower yourself towards the floor. To do this without losing your balance, you will need to keep your left foot flat on the floor and place the crossing foot on its side as you lower your body.

● Use your arms to steady yourself as you move into the sitting position. If you have weak ankles or find it difficult to do this, sit down first and use your hands and arms to get into position. The ball of your foot should fit in the crease of your bended leg.

● Once seated, reach forwards with both arms, turning your palms outwards as though pressing flat against a wall. Flex from the waist and reach forwards (not downwards) as low as you can without lifting your bottom from the ground.

inhale   ▶   exhale   ▶   inhale   11

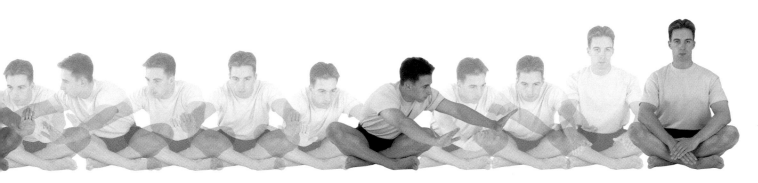

● You will feel a stretch in the buttocks. Now rotate your body to the right, leading with your arms. Keep your abdominal muscles tucked in and maintain a straight back throughout the movement.

● Now slowly rotate your body back to the centre, lifting slightly from the full stretch as you do so. Keep your arms outstretched and palms facing outwards throughout the move. Feel the stretch moving around the back of your buttocks as you rotate.

● Continue the rotation and reach to your left side, leading with your left hand. Remember to maintain a straight back throughout the rotation.

● To complete the movement, come back to the centre and raise your back to an upright sitting position. Relax your arms, cross your hands and rest them on your legs.

exhale   ▮▮   inhale   ▶   exhale   ▮▮   breathe normally   ▮

seated side adductor

This series of side stretches concentrates on the adductors, quadratus lumborum, and hamstrings. To draw maximum benefit from this stretch, remember to concentrate the body weight over the outstretched leg as you lean forward.

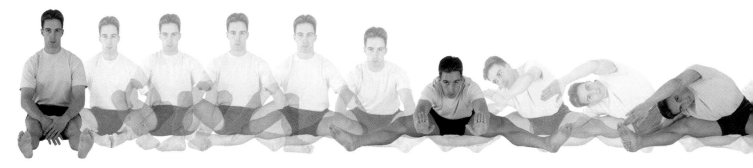

● Start in the seated position, with your legs outstretched in front of you. Rest your hands between your legs. Keep your back straight and hold your head upright.

● Now draw the knees in toward the body, guiding them with your hands on your ankles. Place the soles together, then extend the legs so that they form a 90 degree angle. Extend your arms and press the palms of your hands down on to you shins.

● Now bring the arms together and lean forward, flexing from the waist. Reach forward and push the palms of your hands out flat to stretch the quadratus lumborum muscles. Now slowly begin to rotate to the right side.

● Grasp the sole of your right foot with your right hand and reach your left hand toward the tips of the toes of the right foot. Push this stretch as far as you can. You will feel a stretch along the left side of your body and in the underside of your right leg.

■   **inhale**   ▶   **exhale**   ‖   **inhale**   ‖

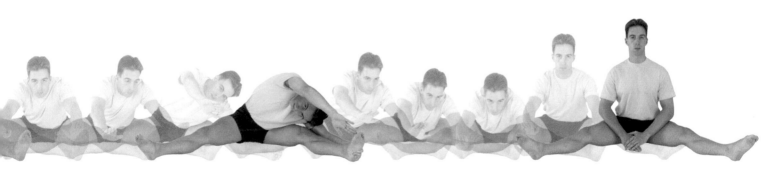

● Now rotate your body to the left side while continuing to reach forward with your palms reaching out. Repeat the stretch on the left side.

● Grasp the sole of your left foot with your left hand and reach your right hand toward the tips of the toes of the left foot. Push this stretch as far as you can. You will feel a stretch along the right side of your body and in the underside of your left leg.

● While holding the stretch, make sure that your body weight is focused above the outstretched leg rather than on the inside or outside of the leg. Release the stretch and rotate your body back to the center, all the time reaching forward.

● Come out of the position by releasing the stretch and sitting upright. Rest your hands and face forward, with your head upright and your back straight.

inhale ▶ **exhale** ‖ **inhale** ▶ **breathe normally** ‖

lying gluteal and hamstring stretch

This is an advanced progressive exercise that stretches the gluteal and hamstring muscles. You will need to lie on a soft surface, such as an exercise mat, to avoid potential damage to your back.

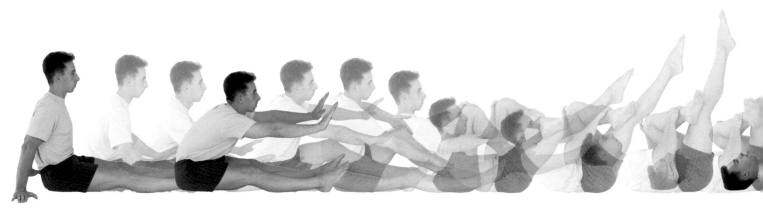

● Sit with your legs extended in front and your hands resting on the floor to support your body weight. Inhale and lean forward, flexing from the waist.

● Continue the forward flexion and reach your arms forwards (not downwards), with palms flat as though pushing against a surface. Exhale and reach towards your toes.

● Now slowly raise your right knee and bring your right hand down to bring your ankle across your left knee. Use both hands to hold your leg in the bended position, your left hand holding the ankle and your right hand gripping the knee.

● Roll gently on to your back. Your left leg should remain extended throughout the backward roll so that when you are fully reclined, your toes are pointed towards the sky. You will feel a stretch in your left hamstrings and your right gluteal muscles.

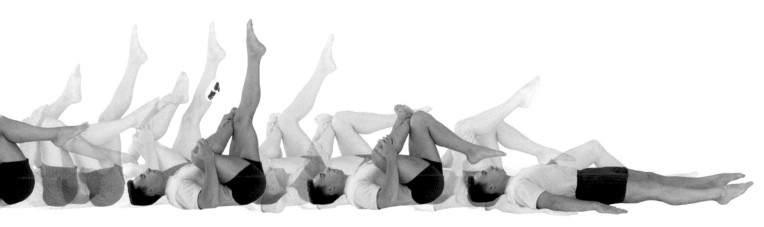

● Now hug the right knee into the chest, lifting the buttocks from the floor. Simultaneously, flex your left knee to 90 degrees and use it to help push your other leg into the body. Hold the hug and feel a more intense stretch in your gluteal muscles.

● Remaining in the lying position, switch legs and repeat the sequence on the other side. Remember not to lift your head throughout the movement, as this can strain your back and neck muscles.

● Keep your right leg extended with toes pointed upwards to stretch the hamstring. Then hug your left knee into your chest and repeat the advanced gluteal stretch.

● After the compression, gently lower one leg at a time to avoid placing unnecessary strain on your back. Rest both legs on the ground and relax.

inhale   ‖   exhale   ▶   inhale   ‖   exhale   ■

rolling side stretch *gluteal muscles*

This exercise produces stretches in your torso and gluteal muscles.

Remember to roll your leg across the body rather than lift it, so as to avoid

injury to the lower back, and try to keep it fully extended for a full stretch.

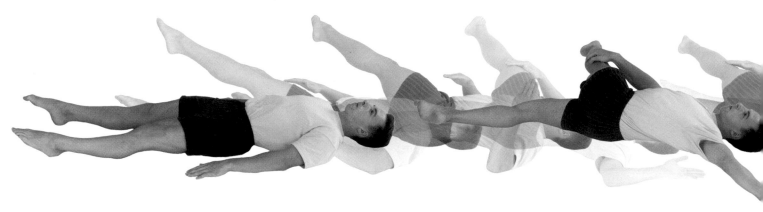

● Start in the lying position with outstretched legs spaced about 12 inches (30 centimeters) apart. Let your arms relax at the sides of your body and press your shoulders firmly back into the floor.

● Slowly raise your left leg, keeping it fully extended. Once it has reached an angle of 45 degrees, roll rather than lift your leg across your body and lower it toward the floor. Hold your leg at 90 degrees to the body.

● Lift your right arm and place it across the left knee, using it to guide the leg across the body. If you find it uncomfortable to keep your left leg straight, flex it slightly at the knee.

● At the same time, raise your left arm, keeping the elbow on the ground, and push it over so that the back of the hand rests on the ground. Fully extend the arm above the head, at an angle of 45 degrees.

inhale ▶ **exhale** ▶ **inhale** 11

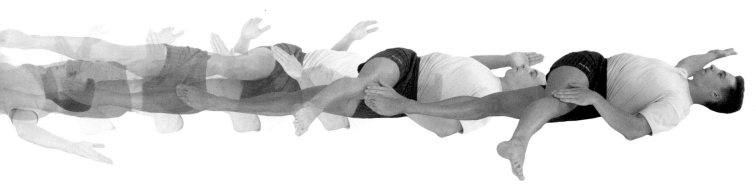

● Hold the stretch in the left leg and keep the breathing relaxed, using long, slow inhalations throughout. Release the hold and slowly bring the left leg back across the body. Now repeat the exercise on the opposite leg.

● Slowly raise your right leg, keeping it fully extended. Keeping the right arm on the floor, roll the leg across the body, and use the left arm to support it as it touches the floor on the opposite side of the body.

● Keeping the elbow on the floor, raise your right arm and push the back of the hand down to the floor. Extend the arm, still in contact with the floor, taking it above your head, at an angle of 45 degrees. Hold the stretch.

● To come out of the stretch, release the leg and take it back across the body. Space the outstretched legs slightly apart and bring both arms down to your sides. Exhale fully to relax the body.

| exhale | ▶ | inhale | ▶ | exhale | ▶ | breathe normally | ❚❚ |

cat into cow

lower back and abdominals

The Cat is one of the most basic yoga positions. This progressive
movement will improve spinal flexibility and stretch the abdomen,
lower back and hip flexors. The sequence finishes in preparation
for the Cow pose (see pages 108–109).

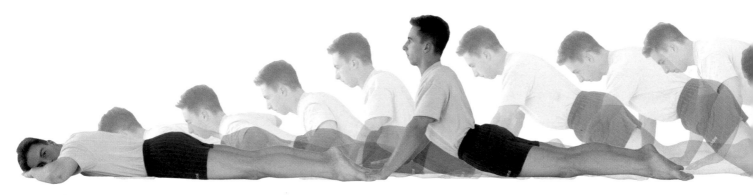

● Lie flat on the floor with your legs outstretched and your head resting on your hands. Slide your hands out from under your body so that they are roughly shoulder width apart, with your forearms flat against the floor.

● Now gradually raise your head and push against the floor with your hands to slowly lift your chest from the floor. Keep pushing until your arms are fully extended and your head is upright and facing forwards. You will feel a stretch in your abdomen.

● Gradually raise your hips from the floor. Walk your hands backwards towards the knees, keeping your back straight throughout. Continue the movement until you are kneeling on all fours and your hands are in line with your shoulders.

● All your weight should now be on your hands and knees. Continue to walk your hands backwards towards your knees until they are just a few centimetres apart and the back is arched upwards in the Cat pose.

■ **inhale** ▶ **exhale** ‖ **inhale** ▶ **exhale** ▶

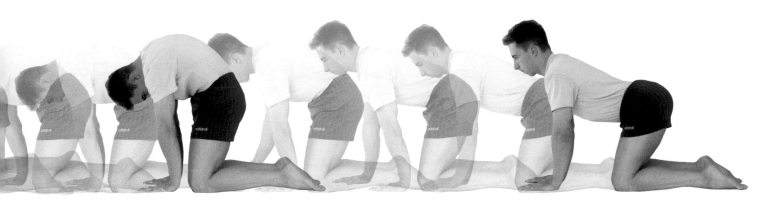

● Hold the pose. You will feel a stretch in your lower back. Now slowly walk the hands away from the knees to straighten the back and release the tension.

● Continue to walk the hands forwards until you have achieved the inverse pose, with your back arched downwards. The inverse arch will help counterbalance the skyward arch and remobilize the spinal fluid in the opposite direction.

● Accentuate the arch in the small of your back. Keep your head up and your tailbone raised to achieve a full arch. Hold the pose and feel a stretch along the spine.

● Now release the pose and return to kneeling on all fours with your back straight and back muscles relaxed. If you wish, you can repeat this sequence two or three times to increase spinal flexibility.

inhale **II** **exhale** ▶ **inhale** ▶ **exhale** **II**

cow into hip flexor

spine, abdominals and hip flexors

This progressive movement continues from the Cat exercise (see pages 107–108). The sequence will stretch your lower back, improve spinal flexibility, and relieve lower back tension, as well as flatten your stomach by flexing the abdominal muscles.

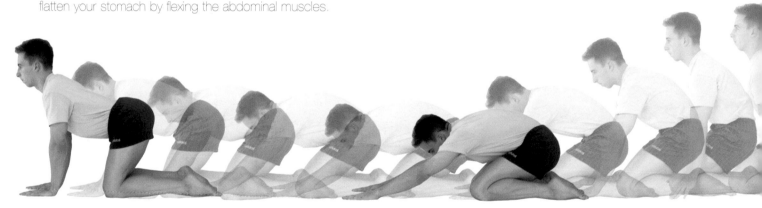

● Start this exercise as you finished the Cat sequence, kneeling on all fours with your hands roughly in line with your shoulders and your back straight and level with the floor.

● Flexing at the knees, gradually lower your hips toward your heels, stretching your back, shoulders, and arms as you do so. Extend your arms and point your fingers away from the body. Hold the stretch.

● Slide your hands backward toward your knees and slowly raise your torso into an upright seated position. Bring your hands on finger tips past your legs and sit upright. Push your chest forward.

● Continue to slide your hands backward until they are level with your feet and your buttocks are resting on your heels.

| inhale | exhale | inhale | exhale |

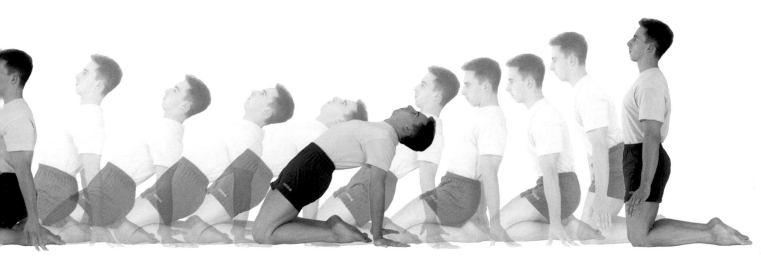

● Move your hands back behind your feet and rest your palms flat on the floor. Arch your chest upward and take your body weight on your arms. Slowly roll the head back so that your chin points upward at 90 degrees to the floor.

● Gently flex your hips and pelvis forward to gain a full stretch. Hold the pose. You will feel a stretch in the abdomen and hips.

● Release the stretch. Supporting yourself on your hands, lower your hips and bring your chest forward to straighten your body. Return to an upright, seated posture with your buttocks resting on your heels.

● Now lift your body from the knees, leaning forward to come out of the seated position. Finish kneeling upright, with your arms relaxed, your back straight, and your head facing forward.

inhale   ▶   **exhale**   ‖   **inhale**   ▶   **breathe normally**   ■

kneeling hip flexor *and quadriceps*

This series of stretches offers a more intensive hip flexor than the one featured on pages 22–23. The sequence will stretch the quadriceps (anterior thigh muscles) and hip flexors. Do this stretch on an exercise mat to avoid damaging your knee joints.

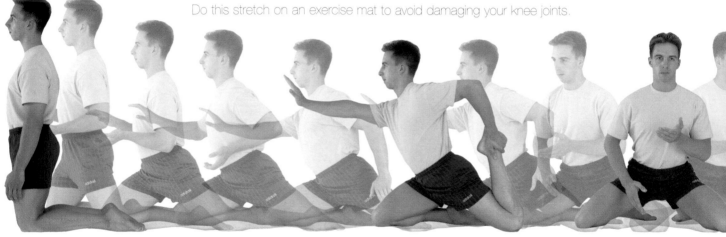

● Start this exercise from the raised kneeling position, with your hands relaxed at the sides and your chest and head facing forwards.

● Now slowly extend your left leg backwards, sliding the knee along the ground. Keep the hips square and the body weight centred to avoid unbalancing during this movement.

● As your leg slides backwards, slowly reach forwards with your right arm, with the palm facing forwards. Reach back with the other hand towards your left foot. Keep your head facing forwards and your hips square throughout the movement.

● Grasp the foot of the extended leg as it bends to a 90 degree angle. Pull the left foot to within six to eight centimetres (two to three inches) of the body; any closer will compress the knee joint. Drawing the leg towards the body will work the quad muscles.

■   inhale   ▶   exhale   ‖   inhale   ▶

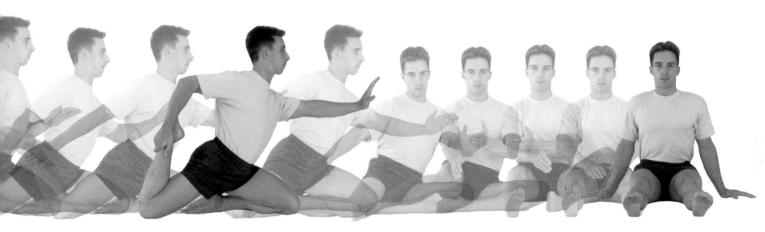

● Release your grip on the left ankle and allow the foot to return to the floor. Now revolve your body to face to the left. Extend your right leg backwards and practise the sequence on this side.

● Reach forwards with your left hand, grasp your right ankle with your right hand, and perform the stretch. Remember not to sit on the bent leg, but to keep your hips square and your body weight centred.

● Release the stretch. Draw the leg back under the body, keeping the torso straight. Keep your arms to the front for balance and rotate the body so that you are facing forwards.

● Sit with legs outstretched and feet facing forwards. Move your hands to your sides and rest them flat on the floor. Relax and breathe deeply.

exhale ▶ **inhale** ❚❚ **exhale** ▶ **breathe normally** ❚❚

crab *hip flexors, abdominals, spinal mobility*

This is an advanced sequence that will stretch and compress your spine,

hip flexors, and torso muscles through two counterposed movements.

The second part of the movement—the Crab pose—increases strength,

spinal mobility, and the flexibility of the nervous system.

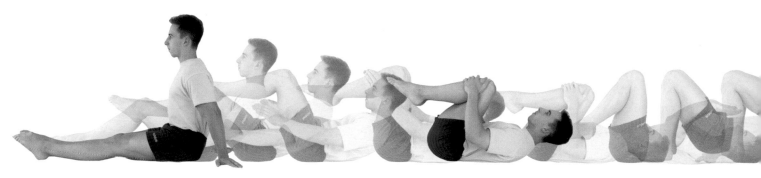

● Begin by sitting upright on the floor with your legs extended forward and your arms at your sides supporting your body weight.

● Begin to roll your body backward in a smooth flowing movement—do not try to hold the movement stage by stage. As you roll, raise your knees and bring your arms out from the sides so that the two meet as your back becomes flat against the floor.

● Grasp your shins just below the knees and pull your legs inward to arch your spine. Hold this pose briefly. You will feel a stretch along the spine.

● Now rest your head on the floor. Release the knees and move the soles of your feet to rest flat on the floor. Simultaneously, reach your hands backward and place them with palms flat on the floor either side of your head and in line with your feet.

■   **inhale** ▶   **exhale** ❚❚   **inhale**   **exhale** ▶

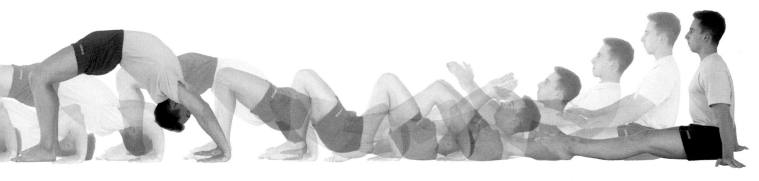

● Inhale and begin to lift your hips from the floor. Continue the movement, pushing with your palms and heels to raise your body into the air, so that the hands and feet take your body weight.

● Hold the crab pose for a few breaths. You will feel a stretch in your hips and abdominal muscles.

● Now gently lower yourself back toward the ground by walking your feet away from your body. Be careful not to compress the spine or strain the wrists by moving too quickly.

● Lying flat with the soles of your feet on the floor, slowly raise your upper body, crossing your hands in front of your chest for balance. Return to the upright sitting position, with your hands by your sides and your palms flat on the floor.

inhale   ‖   exhale   ▶   inhale   ▶   breathe normally   ‖

seated neck stretch

This sequence will stretch your neck muscles (the trapezius and sternocleidomastoid) and relieve tension in the shoulders and neck.

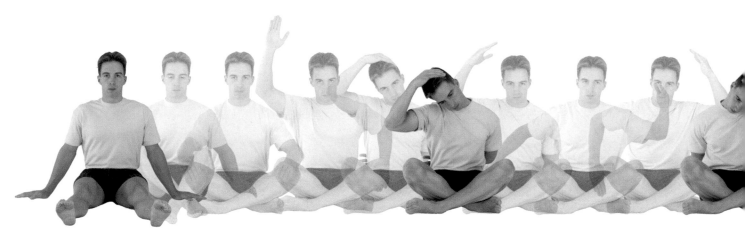

● Sit down on the floor with your legs outstretched in front and the palms of your hands resting flat on the floor at your sides. Slowly begin to bring your knees in towards the body.

● Tuck your right leg under your left and cross your legs just above the ankles. Shuffle your bottom in closer to your legs. Raise your right arm above your head and take your other arm behind and across the small of the back to rest.

● Bring your raised hand over the head and grasp the left side of your crown. Relax your neck muscles and gently pull down with the hand, keeping your body upright. Do not pull your whole upper body, but keep the movement isolated to the neck.

● Release the head, switch over hands and repeat the process on the other side, remembering to keep your neck relaxed throughout. Your supporting arm will keep the shoulder down, ensuring a longer stretch.

■   **inhale**   **exhale**   ▶   **inhale**   ❚❚   **exhale**   ❚❚

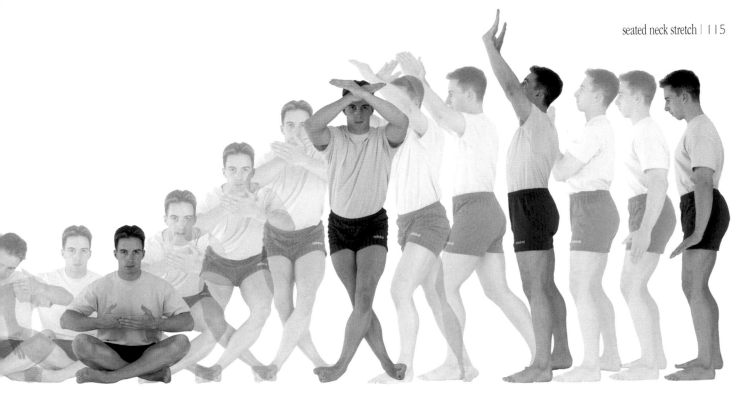

● Now bring both arms around to the front of your body and cross your hands in front of your chest. Slowly raise your bottom from the floor, leaning forward as you do so to maintain balance.

● Continue to raise your bottom from the floor. Throughout the move lean forward to keep your body weight centred. This will place some pressure on your ankles and you may need to put one of your feet flat on the floor to complete the move.

● Now rotate your body to one side and raise your arms above your head, reaching up towards the sky with palms facing outwards.

● Stand with your feet spaced roughly shoulder width apart, bring your arms down to your sides and lower your head.

inhale ▶ exhale ▶ inhale ▶ exhale ■

standing shin stretch *muscles*

This exercise stretches the tibialis anterior and extensor digitorum longus muscles in the shins by dorsiflexing the foot against the floor. There are two movements, which stretch the shins of both left and right legs in succession.

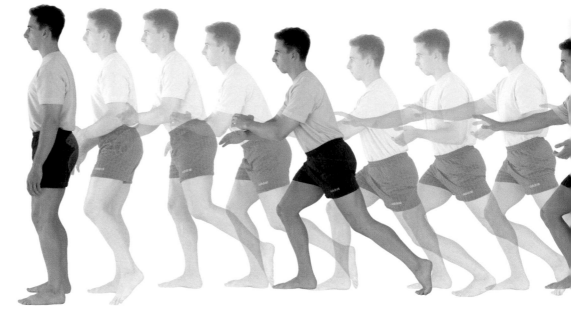

● Stand upright with your knees soft and hands relaxed at your sides. Raise your left foot from the ground and step backward.

● Keep your hands in front of your body to help maintain balance as you extend your leg backward.

● Extend your leg behind as far it feels comfortable to do so. Bend your right leg at the knee to provide support. Keep your arms out in front, crossed at the wrists, and use them to help maintain balance.

● Raise the left foot on to the toes then over on to the flat of the foot. Take a deep breathe. Part your hands and reach your right arm forward to counterbalance the movement of the legs. Keep your hips square throughout the movement.

■ **inhale**　　　　　　**exhale**　　▶　　**inhale**　　　　　　▶　　**exhale**　　　　　▶

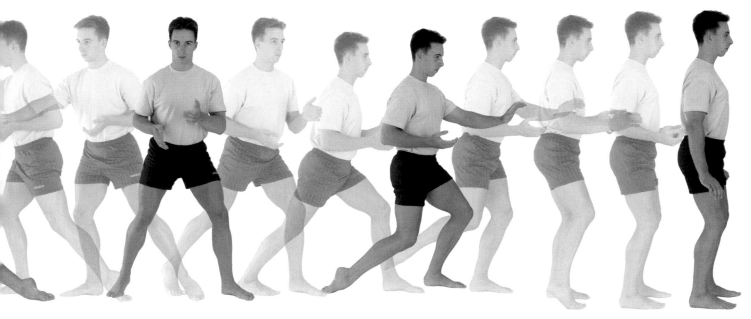

● Flexing at the knee, let your body push your left leg downward while holding the weight on your supporting leg. You will feel a stretch along your shin. Hold the pose for a moment.

● Now withdraw your leg and rotate your body around to perform the stretch on the other side. Keep your feet flat when rotating.

● Remember to inhale when extending your left hand forward to counterbalance the stretch in your right leg. Keep your hips square throughout the stretch and take your weight on to the supporting leg.

● Now return to the upright standing position, with knees soft and arms relaxed at the sides. Breathe deeply.

inhale ‖ **exhale** ▶ **inhale** ‖ ▶ **breathe normally** ▬

standing spine rotation
obliques and abdominals

This is a basic exercise that stretches all the muscles of the torso – the lower back, obliques, abdominals and intercostals. Stretching these muscles will help improve the flexibility of your upper body.

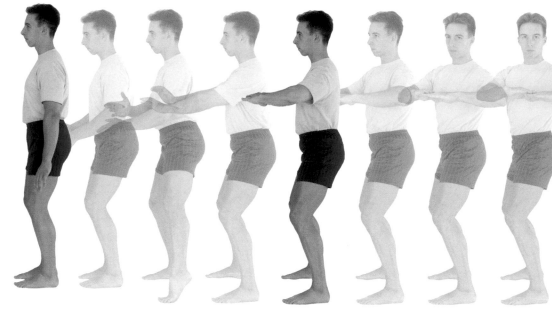

● Stand upright with your feet facing forwards and spaced roughly shoulder width apart. Keep your knees soft and do not lock the joints.

● Slowly bring your hands out to the front of your chest. Bend your elbows and extend them so that they are parallel to the floor. Place one hand on top of the other so that they are crossed at the wrists.

● Bend slightly at the knees and maintain a straight and upright back. Holding your arms steady, rotate the upper body from the waist to your left side. Turn your head in rotation with your body.

● Keep your hips facing forwards throughout the rotation to ensure that all the movement is in the muscles of the upper body. Your hips, knees and feet should form a sturdy base for the rotation.

inhale ▶ **exhale** ▶ **inhale** ▶

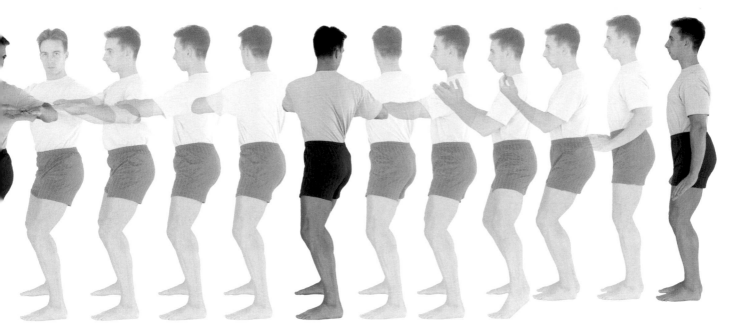

● Continue the stretch as far as possible without turning your hips. Turn your head as far as you can to attain a stretch in the neck. Keep your knees soft and your feet facing forwards. Hold the pose briefly.

● Now release the stretch and rotate the body to the opposite side. Take the movement slowly to avoid damaging your spine or back muscles.

● Repeat the stretch, remembering to keep your feet facing forwards and your hips square throughout.

● Now return your body to the starting position, bring your feet together and lower your arms back to the sides of your body. You can repeat this exercise until tired.

exhale   II   ▶   inhale   II   exhale   ▶   breathe normally   ■

standing side bends

obliques and pectorals

This exercise consists of two movements: the first works the oblique muscles down the side of the torso, and the second stretches the pectoral muscles.

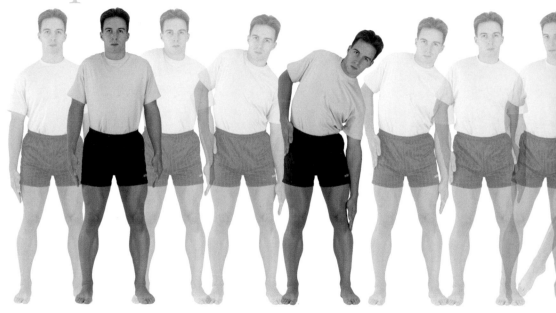

● Stand upright and face forward, with your knees locked and your arms straight at your sides with fingers pointing downward. Your lower body should provide a firm base for performing this exercise.

● Pull both shoulders upward to bring the body upright. To begin the movement, raise your right shoulder and simultaneously let your left shoulder drop downward. Keep your hips and legs square and steady.

● Continue to drop your shoulder and slide your hand down the side of your body toward your knee. Bring your opposite arm up the side of the body to waist height. Remember not to lean forward while bending, but make sure that the bend is sideway.

● Drop your shoulder as far as your can, keeping your head facing forward. Hold the position briefly. Now raise your left shoulder, bring your arms level, and return to a normal standing posture.

■   **inhale**   ▶   **exhale**   ▶   **inhale**   II

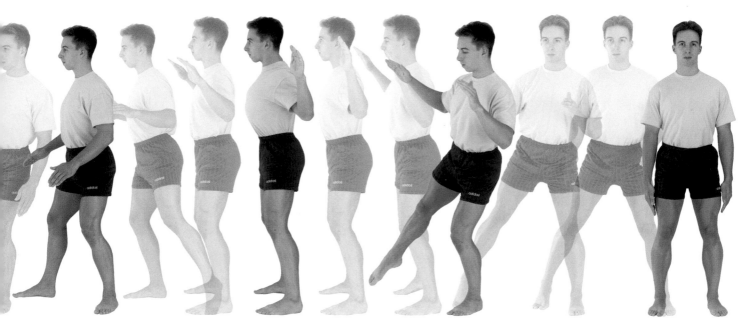

● To do the second part of this move, step to one side and raise both hands with palms facing outward. Keep your legs shoulder width apart and stay soft at the knees.

● Continue to raise your hands. Rotate your forearms back and bring your palms flat and facing outward so that they are level with your shoulders. Push your shoulders back and thrust your chest forward while keeping your lower body rigid.

● Exhale and hold the pose briefly. Now lower your arms, relax your knees, and return to a standing upright posture with your feet approximately shoulder width apart.

● Now repeat the side bend and shoulder stretch on the opposite side. Remember to keep your hips and legs square and steady throughout.

exhale ▶ inhale ‖ exhale ‖ breathe normally ■

standing full leg stretch

hamstrings, adductors and hip flexors

This is an intense adductor stretch that requires great strength in both adductors, hip flexors and the hamstrings of the supporting leg. The leg extension requires a lot of practice; the beginner should not attempt a full raise, but should aim to hold the leg just below waist height at first.

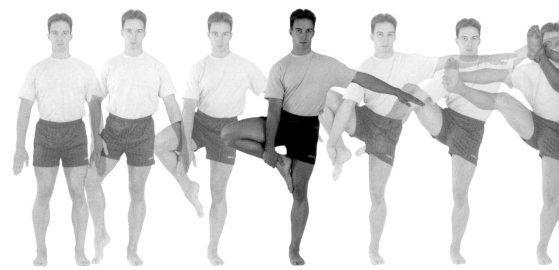

● For safety, when doing this stretch do not force the leg any higher than feels comfortable. Begin the exercise standing upright, with your feet spaced shoulder width apart and facing forwards. Slowly lift your right leg, shifting your weight to your left side.

● Lift your leg with the sole of your foot coming inwards towards your thigh. Reach down to grasp your ankle with your right hand. Keep the other arm extended to remain steady and maintain balance.

● Hold the sole of your foot so that it is resting against the inside of the opposite thigh, just above the knee. Now slowly extend the leg away from the body, using your hand to aid a smooth extension.

● Take the leg out to its full extent and grip the sole of the foot to bring the leg up to about head height. Concentrate on straightening the leg before reaching up for a greater angle. You will feel a stretch along the inside of your extended thigh.

■   inhale   ▶   exhale   ▶   inhale   ▶

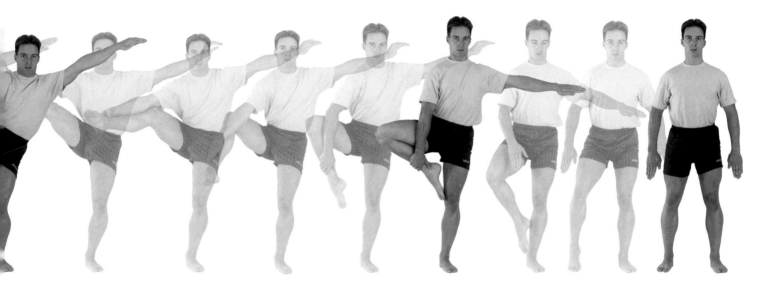

● Exhale and hold the pose. At full stretch push your hips and chest forward. To maintain balance, lean your body slightly to the left with your left arm extended. Do not let the standing leg lock, but remain flexible.

● If you are holding your leg at waist height the guiding hand should be around the ankle; if you have achieved a higher raise, hold the outside of the raised foot.

● Gently lower your leg, using your hand to aid a smooth movement. Use your other arm to maintain good balance and keep your standing leg soft at the knee for flexibility.

● Return to the standing position, with your arms relaxed at your sides. Now repeat the stretch on the other leg, remembering not to cause injury by forcing an excessive extension.

xhale　　**II**　　　**inhale**　　▶　　**exhale**　　▶　　**breathe normally**　　■

closing rotation
latissimus dorsi, quadratus lumborum

This exercise is similar to the Standing Rotation on pages 90–91. It involves a flowing movement that hyperextends and hyperflexes the spine and stretches the quadratus lumborum (lower back), latissimus dorsi, and the hamstrings.

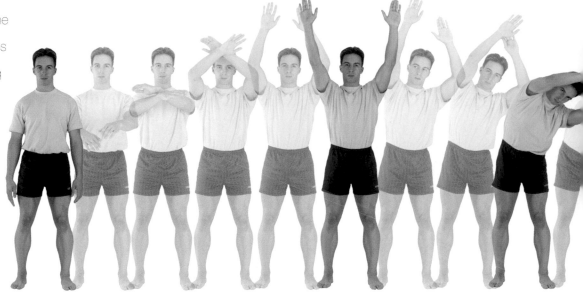

● Stand with your feet roughly shoulder width apart and your arms hanging loosely at your sides. Keep your legs soft at the knees.

● Inhale and slowly raise your arms and cross them in front of your chest. Continue to raise your hands and cross them at the wrists as they pass your face. Move the arms in an upward, expanding movement.

● You should be fully inhaled as your hands reach head height. Reach your hands up toward the sky, facing your head upward as you do. Exhale as your hands extend and briefly hold the pose.

● Lean to your left, flexing from the waist. Grasp your right hand with your left hand to help pull your body downward in a gradual rotation. Pull your leading arm straight to gain an elbow extension. This will stretch your latissimus dorsi muscles.

■   inhale   ▶   exhale   ‖   inhale   ‖

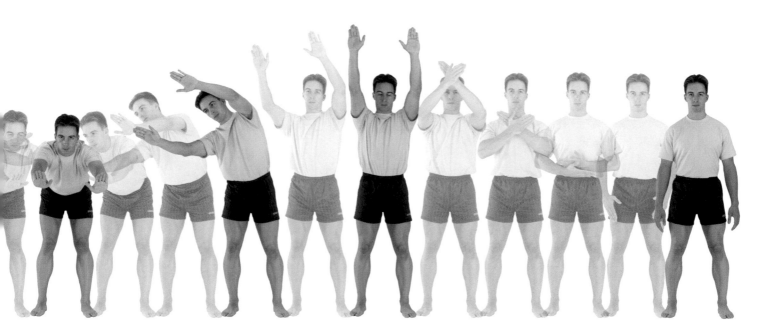

● Continue the downward rotation by pulling your right arm with your left hand and maintaining an elbow extension. Gradually move into a forward rotation. Part your hands, keeping the palms facing outward, reach forward and exhale.

● At the lowest point of the rotation, you will feel a stretch in your hamstrings. Stick out your buttocks to ensure that your back remains straight. Do not let the body slouch.

● Reverse the movement to continue the rotation upward to your right in a shoulder flexion. Keep your hands roughly shoulder width apart and reach skyward to achieve a full stretch in the latissimus dorsi. Inhale as you reach upward.

● Lower your arms, pulling the hands downward and crossing them in front of your chest in a single flowing movement. Bring them back to your sides and relax your body.

exhale   II   inhale   exhale   ▶   inhale   II   breathe normally   ■

index

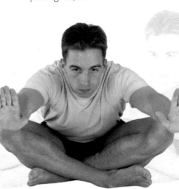